Marijuana &AIDS:
Pot, Politics &
PWAs in America

Written & Compiled by
R.C. Randall

GALEN PRESS
Washington, D.C.

Library of Congress Catalogue Card Number: 91-077140

ISBN: 0-936485-07-8 Soft Cover

Author: Robert Carl Randall, 1948 -

CATALOGUE KEY WORDS: Marijuana; AIDS; HIV; Medicine; Law; Drug Law; Alternative Therapies.

First Printing - November, 1991
Printed in the United States of America

Galen Press
P.O. Box 53318
Temple Heights Station
Washington, D.C. 20009

Marijuana &AIDS:
Pot, Politics & PWAs in America

TABLE OF CONTENTS

IV. LEGAL ACCESS TO MARIJUANA

This chapter contains the paperwork developed by the
Marijuana·AIDS Research Service (MARS) which has been used
by PWAs to obtain legal access to marijuana from the Food and
Drug Administration.

V. APPENDICES

Decision of the Florida Court of Appeals in *Florida v. Jenks*,
overturning the lower court's conviction.

A Parable Of The People Of The Blue Planet

By Michael Aldrich

In the beginning, the people of the blue planet developed a natural bodily defense against the terrifying disease spirits who inhabited their world. This protection, which they called "the immune system," was all that allowed them to live in their harsh and beautiful environment.

From time beyond memory, people used natural herbs, plants and flowers to assist the body in staving off the progression and pain of disease spirits. The jungles and mountains, deserts and plains, oceans and streams of the blue planet were rich in remedies to combat illness and death.

Gathering, growing, and learning to use these natural resources was called "medicine." This knowledge enabled the people to grow into tribes, societies and civilizations.

In most of these societies, people grew medicines in their own family gardens, and the tribal elders passed down the wisdom of preparing and using these remedies, father to son, mother to daughter, generation unto generation.

After many thousands of years, subgroups broke off from the mainstream of traditional medicine and declared that they, and they alone, would have the right to make medical decisions for the people. These groups were called doctors, pharmaceutical companies, and government agencies.

These new groups realized they wouldn't profit from the natural remedies that people could grow themselves, so they organized and took medicine out of the hands of the people. This was called "professionalism."

First, they declared that the medicines people had used for thousands of years were really "dangerous drugs" that caused violence, insanity, and death. They passed laws declaring only "qualified" doctors could prescribe these drugs, and only licensed pharmaceutical companies that followed all the regulations imposed by government agencies could manufacture or dispense them.

Then other groups, called police, preachers and politicians, moved in and said that not even doctors could prescribe these ancient remedies to the people. Doctors who did so were harassed, arrested, and prosecuted as criminals. Only the police, preachers and politicians who knew nothing about medicine would have the right to say which drugs had medical value and which did not.

"Mostly not," they decreed, and they removed all the traditional knowledge from their official medical books. The newspapers and mass media waged crusades against the old medicines, called them names like "Assassin of Youth" and "Weed with Roots in Hell." It soon became necessary for any politician who wanted to gain office to clamor loudly for an ever-harsher "War on the Old Medicines."

And the pharmaceutical companies, unable to patent or profit from the old medicines, synthesized powerful new drugs which they sold to the people at enormous prices. The politicians set up elaborate bureaucracies to ensure that only those new drugs could be marketed and prescribed, so the companies could make billions of dollars and pay huge taxes, so the government could spend billions of dollars on law enforcement to keep people from using the old medicines.

Any of the people who tried to use the old medicines were arrested and put in jail. Their homes and properties were confiscated, their children taken away. And the police, preachers and politicians prospered and multiplied.

And the malevolent spirits of disease and death, which had once been held off by the old medicines, spread across the face of the blue planet.

And there arose a new disease, more dreadful than the planet had ever known. This new disease interfered with the immune system. It invaded the immune system cells and changed them so that instead of manufacturing more cells to fight off diseases, the body produced more diseased cells.

The people of all tribes and societies, the people of entire continents, the people of the blue planet itself were threatened with extinction. In the face of the worst epidemic in history, the policy of the government became genocide. "Let Them Die — They Brought It On Themselves."

And the people suffered greatly.

But the people had not forgotten the wisdom of their ancestors. Against the laws of their governments, against the cruel tyrannies of police, against the profiteering of pharmaceutical companies, against the professionalism of doctors, against the obfuscations of political bureaucrats, the people revived the use of the old medicines.

As their tribal elders had taught, the people began growing their own herbs, plants and flowers, preparing their own remedies against the *ravages of the new disease spirit. When they could not grow their own, desperately ill people went out on the streets to buy their medicines from criminals, often at great expense. Some even set up illegal "buyers clubs," importing medicines over long distances and at great risk. For this they were punished severely by the police and politicians.*

But the people persevered. Bravely, they tried to get permission to use the ancient remedies, through the only legal process available. This was called "compassionate use," and consisted of filing endless forms called "investigational new drug applications" with police and other government agencies.

So many applications were filed that the police and government health officials finally decreed that no more compassionate use of these medicines would be permitted. Instead, the people could use the new synthetic drug sold by the pharmaceutical companies under government license.

"But this is absurd," the people cried. "This ancient medicine is not an investigational new drug, it has been used by the people for thousands of years. And the new drug you offer makes us sicker than we were before, unable to get out of bed or go to work or even think straight."

And the doctors, who had forgotten how to use the old remedies, began finally to listen to the people who had not forgotten, and began reluctantly to learn from the people what real medicine was all about.

And that is the reason for this book.

These are real people, and their stories make me cry. They are proud, and brave, and if the word compassion means anything it means that we understand how valuable they are. How ironic, how frustrating, how profoundly sad it is that their opponents are the very government agencies which are charged with protecting the public health. All the legal obstacles, obfuscation, and hostility that comprise the government's response to this deadly disease, cannot overcome the strength, power and beauty of these people. I thank them deeply for sharing their lives, and I read their stories with tears in my eyes and fire in my heart.

Michael R. Aldrich, Ph.D.
California AIDS Intervention Training Center
San Francisco, September 21, 1991

I. INTRODUCTION

Robert Randall provides an overview of marijuana's medical use in the treatment of HIV infection and AIDS; federal policies governing use of the drug; and the introduction of Steve, the first person with AIDS (PWA) to legally use marijuana in the treatment of AIDS.

Chapter One

POT, POLITICS, & PWAs

*"The people who discriminate against marijuana are
not sick and don't have as much to lose as I do. "*

Steve L., First person with AIDS
to gain legal, medical access to
marijuana. October 1989

This book is about the medical use of marijuana by people with
HIV infection and AIDS. It presents the stories and viewpoints of HIV+
individuals who have smoked marijuana—both legally and illegally—
to achieve specific therapeutic benefits. The purpose of this book is
to provide first-hand accounts of how marijuana can medically help
people afflicted with HIV infection.

For more than 60 years the United States has waged a war on drugs.
This war—fought on the streets of America's cities and in the villages of
distant countries—is a battle in black and white. To the devoted drug
warrior there are no gray tones. Illegal drugs are bad. Marijuana, these
zealots say, must be eradicated from the face of the earth.

We are now entering the second decade of the AIDS crisis. The war
against the HIV virus is waged in hospital wards and doctors' offices
around the world. No cure is in sight and helpful therapies are rare.
Available medications nearly always involve the use of highly toxic,
outrageously expensive chemicals. In hopes of expediting the delivery of
helpful treatments, AIDS activists, through a combination of negotiation
and protest, have attempted to transform the nation's drug approval
process. These warriors are fighting the "war for drugs." That is what this
book is about.

3

The First Casualty

Let me introduce you to Steve. A thirty-three (33) year old Vietnam vet, Steve worked as a tree trimmer in Texas. Steve had seven years of formal education. Steve also had AIDS.

Steve first telephoned me in mid-October 1989. He was calling from his bed at the Audy Murphy Veterans Administration Hospital in San Antonio, Texas. In addition to the routine terrors of his disease, Steve had been arrested for marijuana. Steve was badly stressed, deeply confused, and working through a lot of hurt. After explaining about his illness and his arrest, Steve calmed down and his reason for calling became clear.

Prior to falling ill Steve weighed 156 pounds. After starting intensive AIDS-related therapies Steve's weight collapsed to 86 pounds. He was skin, bones, and not much else. "Then I started smoking marijuana to keep food down and get my weight up. I'm up to 136 pounds on a good day," he told me.

Steve's story was simple. He discovered that marijuana reduced nausea and vomiting and improved his appetite—the "munchies." To the unintentionally anorexic, "the munchies" can be a life-saver.

For two years Steve had asked his AIDS buddies, the doctors at the Veterans Administration (VA), his private doctors, local Drug Enforcement Administration (DEA) officials, and DEA and Food and Drug Administration (FDA) officials in Washington, D.C. to help him secure legal, medical access to marijuana. No luck. So Steve did the only sane thing. He bought some marijuana. The dealer was a narcotics agent for the local police and Steve was arrested. When it rains it pours. So Steve started asking all the same people all over again. This time he found me.

I asked Steve how marijuana helped him cope with AIDS. Without hesitation he repeated a familiar list:

- reduces or eliminates nausea and vomiting;
- stimulates the appetite;
- eases muscle spasms and chronic aches;
- allows him to stay functional and alert.

"When I smoke marijuana I'm living with AIDS. When I don't smoke and take tranquilizers and narcotics, I'm dying of AIDS," Steve explained. "After the police took my marijuana the VA put me on some mean drugs.

I ended up in real bad shape. I don't have those problems with marijuana, and it works."

Several days later I received a package from Steve. It contained nearly a score of character references affirming what was clear in his voice: Steve was a nice guy living through hard times. There was a clutch of personal, handwritten reflections that revealed a keen, sensitive mind. There was also one color snapshot of Steve and his dog, C.B. I could see Steve played for keeps—a very helpful trait to have when you ask the impossible.

Steve told me to call "Papa Bear," a.k.a., Robert Edwards, director of the San Antonio AIDS Foundation. The former owner of a gay bar, Bear has become, unlikely as the comparison may seem, San Antonio's Mother Teresa. Could Bear help? You bet! He immediately put me in touch with the Foundation's doctor, Graham Palmer, who quickly agreed to help Steve.

By November, Dr. Palmer sent the FDA the first request for legal access to medicinal marijuana submitted on behalf of a person with AIDS. The government can grant individual doctors the authority to prescribe marijuana as an investigational new drug (IND). Steve had already gotten farther than most. Usually doctors are frightened of the drug bureaucrats and few are willing to tackle the arcane rules of this forbidding system. Steve was fortunate. Dr. Palmer, Papa Bear, and his AIDS buddies provided Steve with a vital support network. Maybe he had a chance.

In late November I began calling the FDA on behalf of Steve. Things were going well. The people at the FDA appreciated the importance of a timely response and were doing their best to work it out. When I phoned on Wednesday, December 13th, a friendly, now familiar voice said, "You're going to like today's news. Steve's IND was approved this afternoon."

The National Institute on Drug Abuse (NIDA), which controls the government's stockpile of legal marijuana, was alerted and appraised of Steve's situation. NIDA officials were sympathetic and eager to help.

"We can deliver marijuana anywhere in America in 24 hours. For this we're willing to ship without a formal order form. We'll ship on written, fax, or voice authorization. But we can't send marijuana anywhere without DEA's authorization to ship." There was a sense of goodwill. We were rapidly closing in on Christmas.

The DEA claimed it never received Dr. Palmer's Schedule I registration form; had no record of his FDA-approved request for legal marijuana. A flurry of paper and by Monday, December 18th, Dr. Palmer's second registration packet arrived on a desk at the DEA for processing. The clerk assured me it would take no time at all. "I just enter the name into my computer. If it checks out ok I'll walk this one across the hall. It'll be done by this afternoon. Merry Christmas."

It was going like clockwork until someone threw sand into the gears.

Christmas came and went. Steve, home from the hospital, called to say his marijuana hadn't arrived.

The DEA in San Antonio was suddenly on vacation. The DEA in Washington, D.C. couldn't come to the phone. Bear reported that on the Friday before Christmas the San Antonio DEA told him point-blank that Washington wanted things slowed down. Steve wouldn't be getting his marijuana any time soon.

Why? The FDA had approved the doctor's request, the NIDA was ready to ship. The matter was all but resolved. The DEA's abrupt obstruction of an AIDS patient's access to an FDA authorized therapy made no sense. What could the DEA gain by such a delay? Time. But time for what? To what purpose? Steve, twisting in the wind, was sinking into an ominous twilight; approved but unsupplied.

Caught in the Crossfire

On December 29, the puzzling events surrounding Steve's missing supply came into brutal focus when a reporter called to tell me that DEA Administrator John Lawn had rejected the September 1988 decision of his agency's Chief Administrative Law Judge Francis L. Young. In that historic decision—following nearly two years of public hearings—Judge Young had ruled that marijuana has accepted medical use in the United States and should be rescheduled to allow prescriptive access to the drug. Administrator Lawn had taken more than a year to release his agency's final determination in the matter. Not surprisingly, the DEA rejected the Judge's ruling.

Suddenly the delays in Steve's marijuana shipment became perfectly understandable. Steve's urgent need for medical care was being held hostage to the policy demands of an institution addicted to a catechism of controls. DEA Administrator John Lawn manipulated events, transforming Steve from patient to pawn. Steve was caught in an ideological crossfire.

While FDA was approving Steve's therapeutic access to medicinal marijuana, DEA Administrator Lawn publicly declared marijuana medically useless. It would have been inconvenient for an AIDS patient in Texas to receive FDA-promised supplies of medicinal marijuana the very same week Administrator Lawn planned to deny marijuana has legitimate medical uses.

So Administrator Lawn—or someone very close to him— reached into the bowels of the bureaucracy and put a block on Steve's shipment. What if Steve died while waiting? Hey, that's politics. No one in real power within the DEA seemed to care.

Steve Wins, Others Wait

After six rough weeks of waiting, Steve finally received his first legal marijuana on January 25, 1990. In securing licit supplies of marijuana Steve made history. He was the first AIDS patient, and the first Texan to gain legal access to the government's marijuana stockpile. Steve was also the first patient to receive marijuana through a VA hospital. This is not insignificant. Thousands of para- and quadriplegia patients who might benefit from legal access to marijuana receive their medical care at VA facilities.

Eighteen days later Steve died. Thirty months of battling disease and bureaucracies had taken its toll. No amount of what Steve called his "coping drug" could turn the tide. In truth we never expected it to. Marijuana does not cure AIDS. Marijuana—as far as we know—cures no illness. But marijuana does improve the quality of life for AIDS patients and others. And the evidence in this book demonstrates that marijuana can prolong life by helping AIDS patients cope with AZT treatments and maintain his or her body weight.

The DEA could temporarily snag, but not permanently block Steve's FDA-approved use of medicinal marijuana. But the DEA's end-of-the decade decision to maintain an absolute prohibition doomed hundreds of thousands of seriously ill Americans to criminality or needless suffering.

- Approximately 250,000 glaucoma patients are losing their sight. Each year 7,500 to 10,000 go blind while 200,000-400,000 others undergo risky surgical procedures. Many of these patients might benefit from licit access to marijuana.

- Each year one million Americans learn they have cancer. Six hundred thousand receive radiation or chemotherapy treatments; treatments known to cause severe, often uncontrollable

nausea and vomiting. Marijuana is one of the most effective antiemetic drugs known to man.

- A quarter million Americans are afflicted with multiple sclerosis.
Another 750,000 people suffer from crippling neurologic disorders or paralysis. Current medical treatment is seldom effective
and involves the use of highly addictive narcotics, tranquilizers,
and sedatives. Historically, marijuana's most common medical indication was for the relief of spasm and convulsion.

- Nearly 150,000 Americans have AIDS, and 1.5 million Americans
are already infected with HIV. AIDS often causes catastrophic
weight loss and life-threatening anorexia. Every social smoker
knows marijuana makes you want to eat.

These seriously ill Americans want to get their medical care from
physicians. The DEA's refusal to recognize marijuana's medical benefits
condemns them to unrelieved suffering or criminality for meeting their
legitimate medical needs. As the number of patients who smoke
marijuana grows and the war on drugs intensifies, more and more
seriously ill patients will run afoul of the law, be charged as criminals,
and face trial and punishment.

Steve's Contribution

As Steve and I worked together to secure his legal access to marijuana
it became clear Steve had another goal in mind. Securing legal access
was important, but equally important was informing other HIV+ individuals of marijuana's therapeutic benefits. By making history Steve
made news. His story was reprinted in countless newspapers throughout
the U.S. and the world. One friend in Tokyo sent me a copy of a United
Press International (UPI) news account of Steve's story which appeared
shortly after Christmas.

Local television networks in San Antonio and Dallas covered Steve's
story and conducted interviews with him. Slowly but surely word began
to spread. Steve's funeral—complete with full military honors —was
covered by the press and TV.

Even before Steve received his marijuana I was asked by two publications to write a story about his efforts. This chapter is an expansion of
those articles, which appeared in the *Drug Policy Letter* (February/March
1990) and in *High Times* magazine (April 1990).

Six weeks after Steve's death, on March 29, 1990, the Vice Squad in Panama City Beach, Florida conducted a "routine" drug bust on a small trailer. The scenario was typical—8 to 10 cops, battering rams to the door, guns drawn, occupants terrified, contraband seized—but the result was far from typical and would surely have made Steve smile.

The people busted that day were Barbra and Kenny Jenks. The seized contraband amounted to two small marijuana plants and some scales. The police accused the Jenks of selling marijuana. But Kenny Jenks did not use the scales to measure marijuana. Kenny used the scales to measure his life saving medication, Factor VIII. Kenny Jenks is a hemophiliac. As a result of many blood transfusions he is also an AIDS patient. His wife also suffers from AIDS. They, like Steve, had learned that marijuana can be a big help.

Within 48 hours of his arrest, Kenny Jenks bought a *High Times* magazine. He hoped to find the address of some lawyers who could help. What he found instead was my article on Steve.

A Cry for Compassion

The plight of Kenny and Barbra Jenks only amplified the story begun by Steve. More and more PWAs began demanding FDA permission to medically use the prohibited drug. Thirteen months after Steve's death, in February 1991, a national program—the Marijuana· AIDS Research Service (MARS)—was launched to help HIV+ individuals and their physicians apply to FDA for legal, medical access to marijuana by providing them with the necessary forms and paperwork.

The MARS Project, organized by the Alliance for Cannabis Therapeutics and funded by Chicago financier Richard J. Dennis, has been a tremendous success. Within six months more than 400 MARS application packets were distributed to HIV+ individuals and their physicians. AIDS support groups and organizations throughout the United States reproduced thousands of additional MARS packets. Armed with MARS materials, PWAs besieged the FDA demanding legal access to medical marijuana. These demands terrified federal officials seeking to maintain legal prohibitions against marijuana's legitimate medical uses.

In June 1991, the bureaucrats struck back. Beset by hundreds of requests for medical marijuana, the FDA publicly renounced compassionate access requests and the DEA tried to shut down the federal marijuana-as-medicine program. The Public Health Service (PHS) joined in the effort by announcing that PWAs requesting medical marijuana would be told to use Marinol—an expensive, medically inferior synthetic chemical based on marijuana's most powerful psychoactive ingredient, delta-9-tetrahydrocannabinol (THC). While the FDA promised to provide marijuana to the 34 currently approved patients receiving marijuana (not all PWAs) it said no further applications for compassionate access to marijuana would be approved. The agencies wanted bureaucratic compassion based on a quota system. In effect, the drug bureaucrats were saying the federal government had enough compassion to meet the medical needs of 34 patients. If you were patient number 35, you were out of luck.

Compassion Quotas

The basis for this reckless bureaucratic decision, like the decisions in Steve's case, was not medical, but political.

In a series of stunning interviews, federal bureaucrats publicly admitted they were terminating the compassionate investigational new drug (IND) application program for political reasons. One source told the *Washington Post* too many seriously ill people were asking for help. In a mature, rational, humane world such an outpouring of evident medical need would be reason enough to expand the program. But, in the inverse logic of war-on-drugs politics the rapidly increasing requests for medical help were viewed with suspicion; the patients as the enemy. When push came to shove the drug bureaucrats made it perfectly clear they are more than willing to sacrifice the medical welfare of PWAs to the war on drugs.

In the cold, hard world of politics the bureaucrats had no other choice. In April 1991, the U.S. Court of Appeals ordered the DEA to reconsider its long-standing opposition to marijuana's medical use. DEA quickly realized it would have a difficult time telling the Court marijuana has no accepted medical value while the FDA was being swamped by urgent requests from physicians for medical access to the prohibited drug. When forced to choose between the medical needs of seriously ill people and an out-dated, legally discredited prohibition, the drug bureaucrats naturally choose prohibition.

A spokesman for the FDA stated "we don't want to foster a situation in which it appears that the government is saying ...[marijuana] is safe and effective." A PHS official said providing medical marijuana to the seriously ill "might send the wrong message to America's young people." One message was very clear: bureaucrats were more concerned with rhetorical signals than the health and well being of AIDS patients.

James O. Mason, chief of the PHS, was candidly political and mildly homophobic in his comments that were clearly directed at AIDS patients:

"It puts the government in sort of a tenuous situation to be passing out marijuana cigarettes that can cloud their judgment if they choose to use an automobile or get out in the street or in the context of sexual behavior." Mason's assistant, James Freedman of the Health Policy Committee, was even more blunt when he told one irate caller that the compassionate IND program was being shut down because AIDS patients who smoked marijuana medically would "have unsafe sex" and spread the disease even more.

Public reaction to these bureaucratic efforts to terminate compassionate INDs was quick and furious. On June 24th, AIDS activists shut down the Department of Health and Human Services (HHS) for more than an hour. Then hundreds of patients with marijuana responsive medical conditions deluged the White House and FDA with phone calls.

Politics v. Medicine

This is where the story gets interesting. It now appears that the war on drugs hard liners never informed the White House of their plans to terminate compassionate INDs and end the federal marijuana-as-medicine program. Herbert Kleber, Assistant Director of the White House Office of National Drug Control Policy, was particularly embarrassed by the sudden, unexpected bureaucratic attempt to kill the compassionate IND program. A month earlier Kleber, during an appearance on the *Today Show*, had praised the compassionate IND program and actively encouraged patients to apply to the FDA for help. During his appearance, Kleber also declared "This question is not a policy question, it is a medical question."

Kleber was reported to be humiliated by the FDA's termination announcement. With good reason. The sudden termination means Kleber either lied to the American people or did not know what the drug bureaucrats were up to. To make matters even worse, White House officials could not obtain a written copy of the publicly announced termination order from the FDA, DEA, PHS, HHS, NIDA, or the Department of Justice. In response to the termination announcement, Kleber called an emergency meeting of department heads.

Suddenly the PHS termination order announced on June 21 was, by June 28th, described as a "proposed" policy. The White House ordered the drug agencies to maintain the compassionate IND program. The bureaucrats tried to back-pedal. Chaos broke out among the federal agencies responsible for governing marijuana's use as medicine.

As this book goes to press the outcome of this debate over marijuana's legal availability for medical uses is still evolving. One thing is clear. The involvement of PWAs in the question of marijuana's legal, medical use has dramatically altered and expanded the public debate.

Marijuana and PWAs

Like cancer patients in the 1970s, PWAs quickly discovered marijuana can alleviate the dreadful nausea and vomiting caused by AZT and the highly toxic chemotherapy treatments used to combat the HIV infection. Perhaps more importantly, PWAs also discovered that smoking marijuana stimulates the appetite.

The medicinal use of marijuana dates back more than 5,000 years. Marijuana is one of the first recorded medicinal plants to be used by man. So it is not surprising PWAs would begin to use this highly effective medicinal herb.

As AIDS became an established medical diagnosis, marijuana's therapeutic use rapidly spread. By the mid-1980s thousands of HIV+ people were routinely, albeit illegally, obtaining marijuana to meet their medical needs. While information on marijuana's therapeutic benefits spread quickly through the communities most immediately affected by the HIV virus, there was no public discussion of marijuana's medical use in AIDS therapy.

Steve, the first PWA to stand up and demand legal access to medical marijuana. Steve was convinced that his purpose in life was to tell other PWAs about marijuana's important medical benefits. To those who came to know Steve it was clear he was deeply moved by a desire to inform other PWAs who were wasting away from a combination of HIV infection and AZT-induced nausea and vomiting. He was directed by forces he could not necessarily understand, but which surface in his poetry and writings (see Chapter 2). Steve spent the last months of his life battling drug bureaucrats and seemingly insurmountable regulatory barriers to obtain legal access to marijuana. In the end Steve won his battle for legal medical marijuana. More importantly he accomplished his goal of informing other PWAs about marijuana's medical use.

Barbra and Kenny Jenks took heart from Steve's victory and quickly picked up the standard he had raised for others to see. Kenny and Barbra Jenks soon emerged as the principle spokespersons for the medical use of marijuana by PWAs (see Chapter 3). They would win their court battles and convince the FDA of their medical need for marijuana. They would receive the respect and affection of a nation after their story was told on *60 Minutes*.

The ripples of Steve's efforts also touched another life. Danny, a gay HIV+ man in the Washington, D.C. region, read about Steve's efforts in *The Blade*, Washington's gay newspaper. Danny had been illegally smoking marijuana to quell the intense nausea caused by AZT. By smoking marijuana Danny was able to maintain his weight. Danny, a registered psychiatric nurse, decided marijuana was not merely helpful, but critical to his medical welfare. He began his efforts to secure legal access to marijuana in May 1990. It would be six months before he smoked his first legal marijuana cigarette. On Thanksgiving Eve 1990, Danny became the second HIV+ individual in the United States to receive FDA-approved supplies of marijuana (see Chapter 4).

These four individuals—Steve, Kenny, Barbra, and Danny—share more than a disease and a desire for legal, medically-supervised access to marijuana. Through their efforts to legally obtain marijuana each came to feel a sense of participation and control. They could each see how their efforts aided others with similar needs. The powerful, positive aspects of this feeling are enormous.

Specific Therapeutic Effects

Marijuana does not cure AIDS, but its ability to stimulate appetite can prolong life. Steve L. lost more than 80 pounds during his initial bout with AIDS. Barbra Jenks, within a month of her diagnosis, lost one-third of her body weight. The effect of such drastic weight loss—the wasting syndrome—is devastating and life-threatening. Opportunistic infections move rapidly to take advantage of a weakened body. By maintaining body weight patients can better fight infection. Both Steve and Barbra were able to gain back nearly all their weight after they began to regularly smoke marijuana. Both had fewer bouts with life-threatening infections.

Marijuana also decreases the nausea and vomiting caused by AZT and other highly toxic chemicals. Marijuana's ability to control nausea is particularly effective and relief is nearly instantaneous. Just a small amount of marijuana smoking allows HIV+ people great control (titration) over the delivery of marijuana's effects. Most patients report relief after just a few puffs.

Marijuana also contributes to a patient's sense of well being. Most patients describe this as feeling "normal." Commonly prescribed tranquilizers make PWAs feel "like a zombie." Marijuana calms without necessarily sedating. Marijuana helps PWAs focus on life—not death—

13

and makes it easier for PWAs to continue working and participating in life.

Steve expressed the sentiments of many PWAs, "There is no comparison; when I have my marijuana I usually am capable of doing my chores in my house and in my yard and also taking care of my personal affairs. When I don't have it ...I am unable to even get out of bed for long periods of time."

What about getting "high?" If "getting high" means a PWA can sit down to eat dinner with friends and loved ones or get a full night's sleep, what's wrong with getting high? One of the most consistent comments of PWAs who discuss their medical use of marijuana is a sense of changed perspectives. "Marijuana helps me to feel normal." Instead of focusing on the hereafter, PWAs who smoke marijuana tend to live in the here and now. And here and now is the only life any of us have.

Conclusion

This book presents the stories of Steve, Kenny, Barbra, and Danny and the confluence of events that led to a watershed 18 months during which PWAs realized they are not alone in their medical use of marijuana. It was also a time when PWAs realized they will have to fight the drug bureaucrats for this medication, just as they had to fight for access to other medications.

It was a time that brought out the very best in those who made the effort and culminated with bureaucratic attempts to slam the door on compassionate care. It is a sad commentary that three of the four people whose stories are told in this book were arrested for marijuana possession while literally fighting for their lives. In the near future countless others will face similar trials as hard line drug warriors force seriously ill Americans into the streets—and criminality—to secure a medication that can dramatically improve the quality of their lives and reduce the pain and suffering that accompanies their disease. HIV+ individuals who medically need marijuana are caught in the crossfire of the war on drugs. Some, like those in this book, have managed to win the battle and secure legal access to medical marijuana. But the victories are few, the body counts are high, and the prosecutors of the war on drugs have turned a deaf ear to the suffering.

II. THE PEOPLE

Between January 1990 and February 1991, four people with AIDS (PWAs) gain legal access to marijuana through the Food and Drug Administration (FDA). This section contains their personal writings, affidavits, and press stories about their fight to obtain legal access to the prohibited drug. Also in this section is testimony from federal hearings on marijuana's medical use in which a physician provides an early indication of marijuana's medical use by AIDS patients.

Chapter Two

STEVE

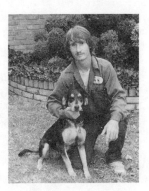

Steve L. & his dog C.B.
October 1988
Inscription on back read, "Hauled two
cords of fire wood to Lubbock, Texas.
With my marijuana medicine
I am not dying from AIDS,
I'm living with AIDS."

October 17, 1989

Dear Bob,

This picture is of me and my dog (C.B. and me). The C.B. stands for Cool Breeze. Fourteen months earlier I was 80 lbs. lighter and laying in bed dying in a comma.

I was given a chance to pull through, but I realized it was hard for me to eat. I was always nauseated and in pain. I also couldn't concentrate on my future because I was freaked out by aspects of Death and Dying.

Certain medications like morphine and Demerol and even Tylenol#3 left me incapable of handling my personal affairs and I needed to get my personal affairs in order in the event of my death.

A friend of mine would come and pick me up at the hospital from time to time and we would drive to the country, smoke marijuana, and talk about things. I found after a while when we did this I was no longer only dealing with the aspects of Death and Dying. I was dealing with the aspects of Death and Dying and the will to live. Now I feel I have more of the will to live and I only consider Death and Dying because everyone should get their store in order, but you should live everyday to it's fullest until you do kick the bucket.

A Bad Day Living is Better Than a Good Day Dead.

Anyway, after I left the hospital I found that as I smoked marijuana I wasn't nauseated as often. I wasn't suffering from pain as often and, when I was, I would smoke marijuana and I was able to overcome or endure the pain and nausea other medications couldn't help me with. Psychologically it helps me control the panic that tries to arise every time they say I'm going to die, including my doctor, family, and friends. Numerous times my doctor has dealt straight with me and told me how long she thought I had left to live. Now she feels I will not live through the winter. I told her no offense but I'm going to try and prove her wrong, again.

Unfortunately I do not have a safe or reliable source to obtain my marijuana anymore. Now I am starting to have medical problems (pain and nausea) and starting to lose my will to overcome my doctors' diagnosis of my life span as well as my illness.

There is no comparison; when I have my marijuana I usually am capable of doing my chores in my house and in my yard and also taking care of my personal affairs.

When I don't have it; it usually isn't long before I start having problems and I am unable to even get out of bed for long periods of time. Most of the time I can't get out of bed until I get help or marijuana.

I'm not trying to get high in my final days. My friends with AIDS are put on morphine and Demerol. After that, eventually most of them started their dying process. These drugs can be fatal. It messes with your dreams and Hell is in your dreams.

I don't want these drugs. I want to use marijuana in what might be my final days. At least then I'm comfortable sleeping or awake and I can feel like I'm alive until the day I die, not dying until the day I die.

Marijuana helps me believe something that some one else said:

I'm not dying from AIDS
I'm living with AIDS

There's a big difference between the two.

I have survived 27 months and 2 days or 824 days with full blown AIDS. There is only one other person in my support group that has lived longer than me and no others have survived the average life expectancy of 18 to 24 months.

Marijuana helps me with the emotional pain suffered as I deal with my friends' illness and their dying. I've lost about 28 friends from AIDS in the last year and a half.

My very best three friends died from AIDS within the first six weeks of this year. My father also died of cancer.

My doctor and my social worker talked to me privately together and told me I was handling it too well and they were worried about me finally snapping from the strain eventually and not being able to overcome whatever problem that would come up.

So they talked me into taking something they said would prevent that.

They gave me tranquilizers. Within a week they said I wasn't making rational sense anymore and decided to give me something else. Every week or two they would change my prescription to something else. Eventually to Halcion sleeping pills.

That was all I could stand. Not only did I come down with a case of meningitis of the brain, but also I suffered from chemical imbalance. Every time I would try to talk to anybody all I did was cry. They even put me on the psych ward for 18 hours.

I asked my doctor to let me out and a friend of mine helped me get some marijuana and within two hours I was home mowing my yard, cleaning my house (washing dishes), and straightening out my personal affairs.

Before I smoked marijuana that day I couldn't even get out of bed for the last six weeks much less talk to anybody without crying uncontrollably.

I'm convinced [marijuana] helps. My doc, friends with and without AIDS are convinced it helps me, and my family is convinced it helps me. Even the sheriff and the assistant D.A. said if I need it and it helps me then I should have it.

I'll always do everything I can to obtain marijuana legally. I've tried for over two years now and it's been painful and frustrating but I think I'm finally achieving my goal.

However, if I'm denied access to it legally I will do everything I can to obtain it, almost any way I can, until I finally get it legally or die. It's my healing medicine as well as my coping medicine.

The people who discriminate against marijuana are not sick and don't have as much to lose as I do.

They probably never tried it and most of them prefer drinking alcohol. I can't drink alcohol. It increases the AIDS virus activity in the body by 250 times. Marijuana doesn't increase the AIDS virus activity. I feel it slows it down so the other medicines are more effective against the AIDS virus. They said I wouldn't last my first 3 weeks with AIDS. Then my doc told me if I was lucky and took real good care of myself I mite (sic) last a year. Not only have I survived 27 months but the first 18 months after my first serious bout with AIDS I trimmed trees, hauled brush, chopped firewood and sold it in Lubbock and San Antonio and I hardly had any problem worth mentioning to my doc. I gained back 80 lbs. and a couple more, and most of my strength, and all my hair.

My doc and many others in the hospital and the AIDS Foundation and my community asked me what I was doing that the dead and dying didn't and aren't doing.

I do marijuana therapy and plan future goals of getting cured and married and raising drug free kids. Not much else except I pray a lot.

Eight months after I got out of the hospital in May of 1988 I cut down a pecan tree that [was] over 200 years old. It was over 100 feet tall and the base was 44½ inches in diameter. I cut the tree down and hauled all the brush and firewood away. I also saved a piece that is 16 feet long and 44½ inches in diameter. It weighed about 8 tons. I loaded it up on to a trailer and hauled it to my property about 20 miles away. A friend of mine has a machine that he's going to use to slice this trunk up into lumber. Another friend of mine is going to build me a coffin out of lumber (the old cowboy style, with wide shoulders and narrow feet).

I feel with all my heart, marijuana has helped me to recuperate from my illness. To regain my strength and maintain my emotional stability to achieve these things I have done in my life since that day in August 1987 when the nurse was holding my hand and she told me that "Steve, you've got to quit talking about those tree jobs you want to do because you will never leave this room alive again."

It was only a few days after that I started smoking marijuana away from the hospital and now the head nurse who was so sure that I was going to die soon is one of my biggest supporters of my marijuana use. She has always told me since then that if anybody can beat AIDS Steve L. can or at least go down after one heck of a fight, with a smile on my face and all my personal affairs in order including my funeral and having my coffin built from a tree I cut down after they thought I would never leave my hospital room again.

Marijuana is good medicine and I'm a good guy with a good dog. The attitude that marijuana helps me to maintain is I have every reason to live for but I can accept whatever is the final outcome. I appreciate everything you can do to help me get my medicine.

Steve
(C.B. & Me)

Editor's note: With Steve's letter there were numerous character references from friends and individuals with which he had worked. There were also several poems which Steve wrote after he was diagnosed with AIDS. They are reprinted on the following pages.

Steve died on February 12, 1990, in the Audy Murphy VA Hospital in San Antonio, Texas. He was buried on February 14 with full military honors. Before his death, Steve had placed C.B. in the care of one of his closest friends in Hunt County, Texas.

Cutting down the last tree

✛

C.B. and me, we're the tree trimmers of Hunt
We're not very big, just a couple of runts
We drive a chevy truck, with tools on the floor
You see us burning brush, during rain downpour

I've been kinda sick and I think C.B. knows that
Sometimes I'm skinny and sometimes I'm fat
We do a lot of work, when I feel good
We spend a lot of time, deep in the woods

Ol' timers tell you, how it should be done
A whole lot of work, with just a little bit of fun
If you make a mistake, and feel awful shame
You know that it's you and no one else to blame

I can deal with that, just leave me alone
Give me a coke and give C.B. a bone
Let us work or let us play
When we're feeling good we don't care what they say

If the time does come soon for me to die
My family and friends will mourn and cry
But God please help C.B. to understand
She is a good dog and I'm a tree trimming man

August 29, 1988

The Day Before The Day After

✛

Living life the way things occur
Saying yes ma'am and saying yes sir
Getting a phone call and being afraid
Sorry Steve you're positive, now you have AIDS

I ask what to do now, as I try not to fall
On the line I hear nothing, nothing at all
I want to be comforted by someone I don't know
She said, "Steve I'm sorry, but now I must go."

Two years and a half, have past since then
Other sick people are now my best friends
Some days are very hard and I try not to cry
As I pray that my friends and I may not die

Life is real different and filling with stress
I'll hang in there ol' buddy, I'll do my best
I believe I will win, I want to be strong
By wanting to live, I don't think that I'm wrong

March 8, 1988

The Visitors Side

✣

Watching the game, from the visitors side
Rooting and yelling, with obvious pride
The home team bench, fresh painted and packed
While over on my side, the paint's peeling, the boards cracked

The home team players are big and react from the yells
Play after play, they're giving my team hell
The score is the Judge, it tells who is the best
The winners have more, the losers have less

My team isn't winning, but I yell and I hope
We may not win, but maybe we can cope
I watch my team intensely and to my surprise
I can see myself, in each of their eyes

There were no mistakes, they didn't really fail
They always got up, after each time they fell
Though they had lost, at the sound of the gun
They jogged off the field, still their father's son

The time's run out and the lights are turned down
The home team left and there's no one around
I realize then with personal pride
Life in this world, is lived from the visitor's side

August 29, 1988

What I think about the cross I carry

✛

Sometimes I'm not in a rush
to get cured
Because certain personal things about me
Have matured
Hope and thanks to the lord
for giving me hope
Indifference to death,
for helping me cope

November 1988

Marijuana
Please let me be me

✢

It's helped me sit and just watch TV
We're perfectly happy C.B. and me
It's helped me to relax and just be calm
You can ask my brother, you can ask my mom

Without it I'll just speed-up or cry
Perfectly honestly, I'd much rather die
I won't kill myself, I'm very much sure
My ambition in life is to hang on till I'm cured

I'll try to be good and not get caught again
But if I do, I'll still be your friend
I don't mean to yell, moan, or whine
But if I slip up please understand and be kind.

C.B. and me
March 31, 1989

Your honor
We're innocent
We're only trying to cope

✙

To PaPa Bear, and Connie and all the bear cub cadets
One way or the other we'll win, so don't you fret
They weren't really ready for this one you know
No matter what happens, I'm ready to show

People with AIDS, need whatever they can get
But they don't need a shove and they don't need a hit
We'll try it their way, the legal way you see
But no matter what happens, we still got to be

If they can't personally help us, or give us a hug
Please leave us alone with our coping drug
No matter what is their perception
Whether legal or illegal, we need our prescription

Now that it's come down to this maybe they'll see
No matter what the verdict, we still got to be
We will always do our best to do what we're told
And if we don't survive this, we'll catch ya on down the road

April 2, 1989

Steve L. became the first person with AIDS to receive legal access to marijuana for therapeutic use. He died on February 12, 1990. He died before his case could come to trial.

Chapter Three

BARBRA & KENNY JENKS

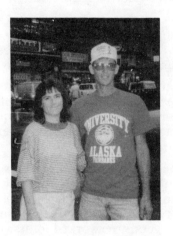

Barbra and Kenny Jenks live in Panama City Beach, Florida. Both in their mid-20s, they fell in love while in high school and married in the early 1980s. Kenny has hemophilia and contracted AIDS from a blood transfusion, probably in the early 1980s. The disease was sexually transmitted to Barbra. They were diagnosed in January 1989.

The following is excerpted from affidavits prepared by the Jenks' for their trial on marijuana cultivation charges in 1990.

Barbra Jenks

If there is such a thing as love at first sight it was me and Kenny. I dropped out of the 11th grade and moved to Panama City Beach, Florida with Kenny in mid-1982. We have lived in Bay County ever since. Shortly after I met Kenny, and when it was clear we were seriously involved, he told me he had hemophilia. He was very nervous and said he would understand if I wanted to leave him.

I had never heard the word hemophilia before and had no idea why Kenny was so nervous and upset. I told Kenny I wanted to be with him and started asking a lot of questions. Kenny told me people with hemophilia are called "free bleeders" and that for "bleeders" even trivial injuries can become life-threatening emergencies. Then Kenny invited me to go with him to the Arizona Hemophilia Foundation so I could talk with his doctors. Kenny clearly wanted me to understand his medical problems.

At the Arizona Hemophilia Foundation I watched Kenny and his doctors discuss his condition. I learned a lot more about hemophilia that day. Kenny also gave me lots of books and articles to read.

Kenny Jenks

I was born afflicted with hemophilia. This disorder, often mistakenly associated with in-breeding, is actually caused by a recessive gene carried by the mother. Female off-spring born to a mother who carries the gene are likely to become carriers of the disorder themselves—but they do not directly suffer the physical consequences of the disorder. Male off-spring, however, while they do not transmit the gene, have a good chance—between 25% and 50%—of being afflicted with hemophilia.

Conversely, males afflicted with hemophilia may pass the defective gene on to their female off-spring, but all male off-spring are free of the defective gene unless the mother also carries the defective gene.

Hemophilia is characterized by an inability of the blood to clot. Commonly called the "bleeders" disease, hemophiliacs are often referred to as "free bleeders." Simply stated, hemophilia represents a critical failure in one of the body's most commonly employed defense systems.

For most people the blood's clotting defense adequately protects the body against all but the most catastrophic forms of circulatory failure. Death caused by massive bodily trauma and a resulting loss of blood is not uncommon. But death caused by blood loss arising from small ruptures, gashing wounds, smashed fingers, overworked joints, and minor impact injuries are extremely uncommon.

Burst blood vessels may cause puffing of the skin or a "blood blister." Running into an object, like the end of a table, may result in the rupture of many blood vessels, the impact area may become "black and blue" and be painful to the touch. The end product is a "bruise." But clotting factors in the blood quickly staunch the out-flow of blood from the circulatory system and allow other cells to repair the injury.

Individuals afflicted with hemophilia, however, lack this critical form of circulatory defense. Due to a genetic defect, the blood of hemophiliacs contains no clotting factor. As a result, even small ruptures or wounds can severely compromise the circulatory system. Untreated, the result can be deadly.

Barbra

I loved Kenny very much and I was not worried by his disorder. The only thing which did worry me was the fact that hemophilia could be passed on to our children. Kenny explained to me that if we had a son the boy would not be a hemophiliac because I did not carry the defective gene. And our sons would not pass the gene along. However, if we had a little girl she would have a 25% to 50% chance of being a carrier of the defective hemophilia gene. While our daughter would not suffer from hemophilia, her sons—our grandsons—could be afflicted with hemophilia. I very much wanted to have a family and this possibility deeply concerned me.

Kenny

My hemophilia was first diagnosed about six months after I was born when I suffered a serious, uncontrolled bleed. Since that time I have been under constant medical treatment.

Fortunately, my father was a career officer in the U.S. Air Force so we were able to obtain and afford the constant care I required.

Throughout my childhood I was subjected to endless hospitalizations. Treatment at that time was fairly primitive. A serious cut or bruise would send me to the hospital where I would be transfused with whole blood or blood plasma.

These hospitalizations could last for weeks or even months and I would receive enormous amounts of blood and plasma just to keep my circulatory system working.

It is fairly easy for people to understand the immediate problem—bleeding to death because blood will not clot. However, a severe bleed has many additional medical consequences.

Uncontrolled bleeding is especially common around joints where blood vessels are stressed. Once bleeding begins in a joint, pressure on the joint, tendons, ligaments, and muscle can rapidly build up. A bleed in the knee, for example, may cause the leg to become swollen from mid-thigh to mid-calf. The skin becomes stretched, extremely tight, and is hot to the touch as blood from a broken vessel uncontrollable flows into the surrounding tissues.

The resulting pressures place tremendous stress on bones and can actually rip cartilage loose. Unrelieved these pressures traumatize nerves. Initially, the result is an acute, intolerable pain that can leave you screaming in agony.

If this type of pressure continues the nerve begins to fail and surrounding muscles start to spasm. These spasms can be slight tremors or violent, uncontrolled contractions that cause the leg to become ramrod stiff and lose its ability to flex.

Over a period of hours or days or weeks this kind of constant, unrelieved trauma can eventually cause the nerve to fail completely. When this occurs the limb becomes numb and the nerve no longer transmits messages from the brain to surrounding muscles. In extreme, but not unusual circumstances, the result may be temporary or even permanent paralysis. The hemophiliac loses the use of the limb.

These kinds of problems were common in my childhood. Even seemingly trivial things, like the loss of my baby teeth, required hospitalization. Physicians at one point pulled six of my baby teeth. The resulting bleed kept me hospitalized for weeks.

I missed school for extended periods of time. Occasionally, I was assigned a special tutor so I could keep up with my studies. On other occasions my teachers would bring work to my home. Several times I missed half of the school year.

Contact sports were impossible. Being hit by a block in football could result in massive internal bleeding—a situation that would be life-threatening.

By the time I reached fourth grade, medical treatment improved somewhat with the introduction of Cryoprecipitate, a frozen blood product collected from several donors. Cryoprecipitate concentrates blood clotting factors and can be directly infused without the need for IV-drip treatment. Cryoprecipitate was much better than the previous IV infusion of whole blood or blood plasma because it placed an emphases on the clotting factor. As a result, controlling serious bleeds became a bit easier.

Nonetheless, I continued to experience severe bleeds, especially around my knees, ankles, and elbows and I continued making frequent, extended trips to the hospital for infusions and treatment. This often involved immobilizing the affected leg or arm by placing it in traction for weeks at a time.

On other occasions I was fitted with a large cast. For example, I would be placed in a cast from my hip to my foot in an effort to allow injured blood vessels, nerves, and joints to repair themselves.

A serious bleed can cause my knee to swell to the size of a cantaloupe. It can take weeks for bleeding to be fully controlled and weeks more before the swelling subsides.

While severe bleeds in the limbs can be painful, crippling and even paralyzing, the most dangerous bleeds occur not in the limbs, but in the upper body, especially the chest and around the neck, head and brain case. A serious bleed in the chest can cause pressure to build up around the heart that, unrelieved, can eventually cause heart failure. A bleed in the neck can stop the flow of blood to the brain. A serious bleed in the forehead can result in massive blood loss and shock. A serious rupture in the brain itself — commonly referred to as a stroke — can be deadly or cause permanent paralysis as massive portions of the brain are damaged or destroyed by uncontrolled bleeding and a build-up in pressure.

Barbra

Kenny told me about the many times he had to be hospitalized because of hemophilia. I wanted to know as much as possible about Kenny's treatment. I continued to go with Kenny to the Hemophilia Foundation where Kenny's doctors taught me how to measure, weigh, mix, and infuse Kenny with his Factor VIII. I wanted to be prepared and know what to do in case Kenny could not transfuse himself or ever really needed my help.

Kenny

Factor VIII is a super condensed form of clotting factor refined from the blood of many, many donors. Instead of simply replacing fluids (as with plasma and whole blood) or slowly increasing the blood's ability to clot (Cryoprecipitate), Factor VIII releases tremendous amounts of clotting factor directly into the bloodstream. As a result, severe bleeds can be controlled much more quickly and with much less swelling.

Factor VIII revolutionized my treatment. After my father retired from military service and went to work first as a border guard and then for the U.S. Customs Department as a law enforcement officer, I received Factor VIII through the base hospital or through the Arizona chapter of the Hemophilia Foundation.

The Hemophilia Foundation office in Arizona is located on the campus of the University of Arizona Medical School in Tucson. The Foundation provides hemophilia patients with information and treatment, gives instructions on Factor VIII, and taught us how to prepare Factor VIII and infuse ourselves.

Factor VIII comes in the form of a freeze-dried powder. This powder must be carefully mixed with distilled water. It is important to carefully weigh out both the Factor VIII and the distilled water so you create a mixture that is not too potent, but is adequate to stem bleeding.

Instructors at the University showed me how to use a scale to measure the Factor VIII and combine it with the proper amount of water. I was repeatedly told never to guess the measurements, but to use a scale to get the proper mix. Precision in preparing Factor VIII is vitally important. A serious mistake could cost you your life.

The doctors also showed me how to infuse myself with Factor VIII. This means I have a scale, syringes, hypodermic needles, and all the other things necessary to self-inject Factor VIII. I was told it was vital for me to have these medical tools handy because bleeds can occur very rapidly. If I am unable to get prompt, professional medical attention then I must be able to cope on my own.

Barbra

After considering all the facts, I knew what I wanted most was to be with Kenny. So, in mid-1982 I left home and Kenny and me moved to Florida. It was a decision I do not regret.

Kenny

Around 1981, physicians at the Hemophilia Foundation began warning me about a new, as yet unnamed disease, that was beginning to affect hemophilic patients.

There are literally dozens of blood-borne diseases. Among the most dangerous is hepatitis, which can injure the liver and, in extreme cases, cause death. About 10% to 15% of patients who contract hepatitis die as a result of liver complications.

Hepatitis is very common among hemophiliacs because they are compelled to use such massive amounts of whole blood, blood plasma, Cryoprecipitate and Factor VIII. While great strides have been made in my life time to improve the safety of transfusions, nearly every hemophilic person I have ever known has contracted hepatitis at least once. I am an exception. I had never contracted any diseases as a result of my constant need for transfusions.

By early 1982, however, doctors at the Hemophilia Foundation were becoming alarmed. They were convinced that an altogether new disease, which often mimicked hepatitis in its early stages, was beginning to sicken and kill hemophilic patients.

I received a letter from the Arizona Hemophilia Foundation warning patients about this new disease. Once I realized the doctors were worried I began asking questions. They told me the disease appeared to disrupt the immune system and that this disruption resulted in a host of what they called "opportunistic" diseases. Opportunistic diseases are generally common maladies ranging from household bacteria to various types of molds, fungi, and viral infections. Usually these ever-present toxins and molds are destroyed by the body's immune system. If the immune system begins to fail, however, even a common cold becomes a life-threatening illness.

After listening to the doctors outline the problem as best they could, I asked what were the chances that a hemophiliac with my history of serious bleeds could contract this seemingly deadly disorder.

They tried to reassure me by saying that the blood supply was safer than ever and that the odds were less than 1 in 100,000 that I could contract this new disease. They seemed fairly confident that most hemophiliacs would not be affected by this still unnamed new disease.

Shortly after these conversations, Barbra and I left Arizona and moved to Florida so I could be close to my mother who lives in Ft. Walton Beach.

Barbra

Both Kenny and I are hard workers. I have worked steadily since the age of 16. I have held a variety of jobs including a full-time hotel/motel housekeeper, in restaurants, and as a convenience store clerk. I have also held a number of part-time jobs and helped my husband run a hot dog stand ("Chicago Dawgs") on the beach during the summer tourist season. Both Kenny and I nearly always worked more than one job at a time.

On a typical day we would wake up around 4 a.m. and go to work cleaning up a bar/restaurant. We usually finished our cleaning job around 7 a.m. Then Kenny and I would go to our regular, full-time jobs. I would go to my motel housekeeping job and work until 4 or 5 p.m. If there was any time I would rush home for a quick nap. Then, around 6 p.m. I would drive to the beach to meet Kenny at the hot dog stand. If the stand was not busy I would relieve Kenny and he would head home for bed. Often, however, business was booming and we would both stay and work until 2 a.m. Then we would rush home, hop into bed, get two or three hours sleep and start over again.

We worked like this six days a week. On the weekends I did not usually go to the motel, but started working at the hot dog stand in the early afternoon. On weekends we often worked at the stand until 4 a.m. I'm one of those people who really enjoys working hard.

We are happy in Florida. Kenny's mother, Alma Dee, lives nearby in Ft. Walton. She and I get along unusually well. We love to visit together and talk. I call her "Mom." It's a great relationship to have with an in-law.

After years of working on the beach both Kenny and I know a lot of people and we have made some real friends in the nine years we have lived in Panama City Beach. It felt good to be part of the community.

Kenny

We settled in Panama City Beach and I worked a variety of jobs. For a period of time I did landscaping work, then I began cleaning restaurants and bars. I often worked one full-time and one-part time job. Barbra is also a hard worker and together we made enough money to live fairly well.

We did have one major problem. Because I have hemophilia I cannot get health insurance and, after leaving Arizona, I discovered Florida does not have a Hemophilia Foundation like the one in Arizona.

This led to serious problems. First, I could not afford Factor VIII, which costs between $500 and $700 per dose. In Arizona the physicians told me "when in doubt, transfuse." During a normal month I would use Factor VIII two or three times. If I got a really serious bleed I might require Factor VIII much more frequently.

Second, in Florida I could not often get Factor VIII to take home. So every time I had a serious bleed I would have to rush to the Bay County Medical Center and wait in the emergency room for treatment. On many occasions I had to wait four or five hours to receive Factor VIII.

This was very costly and didn't make any sense. Even when the emergency room staff finally got around to treating me they usually gave me the Factor VIII, so I could weigh out the proper amount, mix it, and infuse myself. All of this could have been done much more quickly and inexpensively at home.

Barbra

In Arizona the doctors at the Hemophilia Foundation taught Kenny "when in doubt, infuse." If there was even a possibility of a bleed, Kenny should use his Factor VIII and infuse himself as quickly as possible. But in Florida, Kenny could not afford to keep Factor VIII at home. Instead, he had to rush to the hospital emergency room to get a Factor VIII infusion, As a result, Kenny often did without proper treatment. He would get minor bleeds and, instead of infusing, simply hoped the bleed would not turn into a major hemorrhage.

While in Arizona, Kenny had used the Factor VIII infusions about twice a month. Sometimes, of course, if he suffered a major bleed he needed Factor VIII infusions much more frequently. In Florida, however, Kenny cut his use of Factor VIII infusions way back. This concerned me because the less often Kenny used his Factor VIII infusions the more serious his bleeds became.

Kenny

In 1984, I was working as a carpenter and fell off the second floor of a building under construction. I landed on my back and hip. At first I seemed to be alright. I had not broken any bones and there did not seem to be much internal bleeding.

By the next morning, however, my hip began to swell. I phoned my doctor and he told me to get to the hospital as quickly as possible. I went to the emergency room, where I waited for hours before someone could bring me some Factor VIII. After I infused myself I returned home, hoping I could get by with just one shot.

By that night, however, it was clear the bleeding was still uncontrolled. By the next morning I was screaming in pain as pressure on my hip joint rapidly increased. Swelling extended down my leg and my knee joint also began to bleed uncontrollably. This further increased the pain and my leg began going numb as the nerves began to fail.

I rushed back to the hospital emergency room where, after waiting for several hours, I was informed the pharmacy had completely run out of Factor VIII. I had no alternative but to wait until that afternoon when a shipment finally arrived from the warehouse.

By then the bleeding was completely out of control. My leg was spasming violently and the nerves were growing numb. When my doctor realized just how serious things had become he immediately hospitalized me. Despite two infusions of Factor VII,I I was still bleeding profusely.

For the first four days I received infusions of Factor VIII every six hours — double the normally permitted dose — as my doctor struggled to regain control over the intense bleeding. Then I continued to receive infusions of Factor VIII once every twelve hours for the next week.

This intensive Factor VIII therapy eventually brought my bleeding under control. But the damage was very extensive. I completely lost the use of one leg from traumatic injury to the nerves. My knee joint, already weak, was unable to support my weight. When my wife Barbra finally wheeled me out of the hospital the doctor told me he didn't think I would ever walk again.

Barbra

At the time Kenny was hospitalized in 1984, we already owed the hospital more than $45,000. By the time Kenny left the hospital after his major bleed we owed the Bay County Medical Center more than $125,000. There was, of course, no way we could pay such an enormous bill. As a result we could not get credit. So we had to buy everything we needed on a cash-and-carry basis.

Kenny's huge hospital bill was eventually paid by someone we do not know. I discovered this when I suddenly realized we had stopped receiving our regular dunning calls from the bill collectors. I did a little checking. The hospital simply told me all of Kenny's bills had been paid in-full and we were up-to-date. When I asked the hospital to tell me who paid the bill, however, they refused. It remains a pleasant mystery to this day.

I was greatly relieved and deeply touched that someone in Bay County had the heart to think of us and to help us through this very difficult time. It made me feel Kenny and I were no longer "outsiders." We had finally become part of the community.

Kenny

Shortly after this experience, while I was still trying to regain use of my leg, my doctor began telling me about problems with the blood supply. The unnamed disease now had a name; acquired immune deficiency syndrome or AIDS. And AIDS was beginning to kill hemophiliacs.

In an effort to reduce my chances of infection he switched me off of Factor VIII and back to the older form of treatment, Cryoprecipitate. He said that cryo-therapy involved the use of far fewer donors and thus significantly reduced my chances of contracting AIDS. He also explained that AIDS was poorly understood, incurable, and always fatal.

I began reading newspaper articles and listening to television news reports about this new disease. Mostly, however, it appeared to affect only highly selective groups. These included homosexual and bi-sexual men, IV drug users and, for reasons still not clear, Haitians. The news reports mentioned that AIDS was transmitted sexually or through an exchange of dirty needles. Less often the reports noted AIDS could be contracted through transfusions which involved the use of contaminated blood or blood products.

At first I thought little of these reports. I am not gay or bi-sexual and I do not use illegal drugs or dirty needles. I felt confident this fatal disease would never affect me, especially after my doctor had further reduced my risk of contracting this new disease by transferring me back to cryo-treatment.

Barbra

I first heard about AIDS in 1984 or 1985 while watching the nightly television news. At the time I did not pay much attention to the report because it mostly talked about how AIDS only afflicted male homosexuals and Haitians.

I remember the reporter mentioning there were some who feared AIDS was a blood-borne disease and that it might affect the blood supply. But the report greatly downplayed the possibility of tainted blood posed a serious danger to anyone and went on to emphasize the likelihood of contracting AIDS from a transfusion were extremely small. I believe the reporter said it was something like one in 10 million.

Though I remembered the report I did not become alarmed. The news did not seem to affect Kenny and me. His Factor VIII was a pharmaceutically prepared product and I felt certain the manufacturer would do everything possible to protect hemophiliac patients from the possibility of getting a contaminated blood product. If I had any lingering concerns they were quickly overwhelmed by the rush of our busy lives.

I remember seeing other news reports on AIDS, and occasionally read a newspaper article on how the disease was spreading. And I began to realize how frightening AIDS is and how frightened people are of people who have AIDS. But the reports always centered on particular groups of people who got the disease. Fear of homosexuals seemed to be the same as fear of AIDS.

Kenny

Then, in 1987, my doctor informed me that one of his other hemophiliac patients had tested positive for the HIV virus that is the cause of AIDS. He told me I had received an infusion from the same numbered batch as this now-infected man. The doctor told me I should get tested for the HIV virus.

Barbra

We were in shock. Kenny and I discussed getting tested on the way home. In my heart I knew right then it was just a matter of time before Kenny and I were going to get sick with AIDS. But I did not say this to Kenny and, after talking, we decided not to get tested. We were afraid if Kenny tested positive he would lose his job, we would lose our friends, and be subjected to all sorts of harassment from our neighbors.

Kenny

My wife and I discussed the possibility I might be HIV+. The idea was scary. We did not know much about AIDS, except that it was always fatal, and that a lot of misinformation and fear surrounded the disease.

We also knew that several other hemophiliac patients had suffered tremendous social problems because of the disease. Ryan White, a young kid in Indiana, was taunted by other students and thrown out of the public schools. Eventually, his family was forced to move because of the stigma attached to his disease.

Barbra

Looking back on this I realize our attitude—our desire to not know—might seem strange to someone else living in a more reasonable world. But this was happening to us. And it was happening around the same time a young Indiana boy with hemophilia named Ryan White was cursed by his neighbors, beaten by his fellow students, then thrown out of school and eventually run out of town simply because he had AIDS.

And it was around the same time the Ray brothers—three young teenage hemophiliacs with HIV infection who lived in Arcadia, Florida —were taunted by neighbors and voted out of school. When the Ray family tried to fight this hysteria with facts about their disease, they were despised by their community and burned out of their family home.

And, out of the blue, the doctor told Kenny we might have this dread disease.

Fear entered into my life: fear of AIDS, fear of sickness, fear of dying, fear of neighbors, fear of friends. Suddenly, there was no one to talk with. No one to trust. I was just plain scared.

I read all the newspaper articles and saw all the television news shows looking for information on AIDS. Everything I learned only increased my fear. The disease was incurable and there were no treatments. Hundreds, then thousands, then tens of thousands of people were dying from this dreadful disease, yet no one in government seemed to care.

Kenny

The more my wife and I thought about the possibility I might be infected with this same virus, the more reluctant we were to get tested. I realized we had been at risk for years and, if I had received tainted blood, my chances of being infected were close to 100%. If I'd received tainted blood, then the likelihood I'd already passed the virus to Barbra was also extremely high.

And we also confronted the stark reality that there were no effective treatments for HIV infection. While doctors could treat some of the opportunistic infections caused by AIDS, they could not control the HIV virus. As a result the disease was 100% fatal. No one with AIDS lived long.

Barbra

For the first time I came to understand prejudice. No one cared because the only people dying were gay men and IV drug addicts. Why bother to save them? This mean-spirited, vengeful thinking was common place. People blurted it out in the middle of a conversation. Preachers told their congregation that AIDS was God's way of punishing homosexuals, drug addicts, and other sinners. Were Kenny and I sinners?

It was like the Dark Ages with its fear of witches. I began feeling like a leper. A deep foreboding reached into every corner of my life. Kenny and I stopped talking to one another. We never discussed AIDS in our house. Maybe if we didn't talk about it we wouldn't get it.

Kenny

In the absence of effective treatments, and very frightened over how our own community—described even by locals as the "Redneck Riviera"—would react, we decided our best course of action was to just wait and see.

After we made that decision Barbra and I never again discussed AIDS. It became a forbidden subject. News reports only made us more and more apprehensive, but we never discussed our situation or the possibility we might be infected.

Barbra

Every time we went to see Kenny's doctor he told us to get tested for HIV infection. We ignored his advice. If Kenny and I talked about AIDS at all it was while driving home from the doctor's office. Whenever we talked we always reached the same conclusion: we were probably already infected and it was too late to do anything about it. We were too scared to get tested.

In the spring of 1988, I developed a vaginal yeast infection. At first I dismissed it as a typical "female problem." I tried several treatments. Each seemed to work for a short period of time. Then the yeast infection would return.

Then one day around my birthday in July 1988, while my sister was visiting from Arizona, my mouth started to hurt. It felt like tiny needles were being stuck into my tongue. By that evening my whole tongue had turned white. I became alarmed and tried to brush it off. I brushed my tongue and gums raw.

At first this seemed to work. But in a matter of hours my tongue was coated white again.

I went to my doctor. He looked at my tongue and told me I had an uncontrolled yeast infection. I told him about Kenny's hemophilia and about the tainted blood he had received. The doctor gave me a prescription for a powerful antibiotic and wrote out an order for me to be tested for HIV infection at the Bay County Medical Center.

Kenny

At first, Barbra's yeast infection subsided. But soon after the antibiotics prescription ran out the yeast infection in her mouth returned. She developed thrush — a generalized yeast infection throughout the mouth. Yeast also developed in her ears, nose, and sinuses.

I also began getting yeast infections in the mouth.

Barbra refused to return to the doctor. Her weight started dropping rapidly and she developed a constant, hacking cough. We tried to pretend everything would be ok. We never discussed our fears.

Barbra

At first the medicine the doctor prescribed seemed to kill the yeast infection. After taking the antibiotics for seven days the yeast was completely cleared up. Within a month, however, the yeast returned and my tongue was coated white once again.

I returned to my doctor. He asked me if I had been tested. I told him I had not been tested. But I said Kenny had been tested and the test had come back negative. Put simply, I lied. I was panic-stricken. My life seemed to be slipping out of control.

The doctor sternly told me it did not matter if Kenny was HIV+ or negative. I clearly had a serious immune deficiency problem and should get tested. My doctor wrote out a second order for an HIV test at the Bay County Medical Center. Then the doctor gave me another prescription for antibiotics.

Instead of getting tested I took the new antibiotics. After several days the yeast went away. When the yeast did not come back immediately I was relieved, but I didn't feel better. I am usually highly energetic. Now I felt like I was really dragging.

This sense of fatigue grew daily, and my yeast infection returned. Despite my lack of energy I continued working two jobs and never missed a day. Kenny also developed a yeast infection but continued working. We tried to pretend things were normal. Things were far from normal.

In the morning I would wake up, walk into the bathroom and vomit. When I brushed my teeth the taste of the toothpaste mixed with the yeast and caused me to gag. My muscles and joints constantly ached. I stopped making dinner—the sight and smell of food made me sick to my stomach. I eventually stopped eating because of the constant vomiting and nausea.

I wanted to sleep all the time. Then Kenny and I started getting night-sweats. When we woke up our sheets and pillows would be soaked with sweat. I would wake up feeling more tired than when I went to sleep.

Kenny and I stopped talking. We didn't communicate about anything. We were withdrawn, both extremely worried about the other.

Kenny

Between Thanksgiving and Christmas 1988, Barbra's weight collapsed. She went from around 150 lbs. to less than 115 lbs. She felt constantly nauseated and was unable to eat. Her coughing became worse and she was constantly fatigued.

Barbra and I started having night sweats. These are drenching, bed-soaking bouts of sweating that seem to drain energy out of you.

43

I pleaded with Barbra to go to the doctor. She refused. She continued to work.

Barbra

On the night following Christmas I could not breath. I tried to sleep sitting up, but I was gasping for air and could not relax, much less sleep. The next morning I decided not to go to work. I almost never miss work, but for the first time in my life I did not think I could make it through the day. I called in sick at 5 a.m. and arranged for someone else to take my place.

At 9 a.m. I called my doctor and tried to make an appointment. I drove to his office, but he could not see me immediately. Upset, and not thinking clearly, I drove home. Once I got home I did not have enough energy to make it back to the doctor's office. Kenny came home from work around 5 p.m. and found me sitting on the sofa, barely conscious, and gasping for air. He rushed me to the doctor's office. The office was still crowded and we had to wait nearly two hours before I could see the doctor.

I half-stumbled into my doctor's office. As soon as he saw me he became alarmed. He listened to my breathing and heart and asked me again if I had taken my HIV test. This time I told him the truth. The doctor immediately made arrangements for me to be hospitalized and tested. Within two hours I was in the hospital undergoing dozens of tests and being given oxygen. When it appeared my lungs would fail I was placed on an artificial respirator.

Kenny

Barbra was tested in the hospital that evening. The test for HIV infection came back positive. I was tested the following week. My test was also positive. At the time of my test my T-cell count was less than 150—ten times lower than a healthy count. T-cells are the body's disease fighting cells. Without T-cells the immune system fails in much the same way hemophilia affects the circulatory system. Unable to combat incoming infections the body is exposed to horrific, little understood diseases.

Barbra was diagnosed as having *Pneumocystis carinii pneumonia*, one of the most lethal AIDS-related diseases. She was placed on a respirator, then slipped into a coma-like state. She could not recognize my face or hear my voice. She did not respond to touch. If she tried to speak she was incoherent. Often she just drooled.

Barbra

I was given massive doses of direct IV antibiotic therapy. At first I could barely speak and floated in and out of sleep. Then I lost consciousness and slipped into a deep coma. I lost all track of time.

At some point during my coma I had a near-death experience. I entered into a kind of awareness and suddenly sensed I was standing up. Next to me was a shadow and I knew the shadow was me. I was surrounded by tunnel-like blackness, but there were no walls. In the far distance, through a break in the darkness, there hovered a blue-white fog that beckoned me. I saw this light not with my eyes, but with my whole spirit—my whole being. And I knew the light was good. I did not feel warm or cold or any other physical thing. I heard a light breeze that I could not feel, yet sensed it with my whole self.

Without question I knew the light was kind and gentle and good, and that if I reached the light I would be happy—joyous. And as I knew these things the light came closer—but I could not tell if I was moving to the light or the light to me. And I came to realize if I reached the fog and entered into the light I would be forever separated from my physical self, and that my body would die.

There was no alarm or fear in this revelation. Instead I sensed the presence of an encompassing love. My fears and hates melted before the light. Sadness left me, and I felt whole as I have never before felt. I wanted only to reach the light and become the light.

I was about to enter the light when I thought of Kenny and I wondered who would take care of him? Who would fix his dinner? Who would mix his Factor VIII? Who would make certain he received good medical treatment for his hemophilia and his AIDS?

And with the thought of Kenny I came to understand it was not my time to enter into the light. And as soon as this understanding came to me the light began to recede from me and I heard again but did not feel a light wind against my spirit and saw again the shadow that was me. And then I awoke.

I felt a sense of surprise and moved my hands to my face to feel my physical self. I discovered I was still in the hospital, still sick, still receiving massive doses of drugs, still strapped to IV needles and oxygen tanks. When my hands hit the oxygen mask I smiled.

I was exhilarated and disappointed. My body, which had so ached when I went into the hospital, felt less pain and my fears seemed vanished. I knew it was not yet time for me to die, but that when the time came I would be ready, even willing to enter into the light and into the joy within the light. I felt a great peace.

Kenny

This coma-like condition lasted for nearly two weeks. Then, slowly, she started to recover. Her pain seemed less intense, her breathing easier. After nearly a month in the hospital I took Barbra home.

Barbra

I remained in the hospital for many days. When I was alone I reflected on this experience. I tried to make it just another dream. But it was more vivid, more real than any dream I have ever had. Through this experience I learned things I had always known about myself, about my life, about life itself. I had not died because it was not yet time for me to die. I had not died because there was something undone—something I was to accomplish that I had not yet accomplished.

I had no idea what this something was. And I had no desire to go out in search of it. I knew whatever it was I had to do would come to me, would be accomplished without pain. Once accomplished, my time in the physical world would end and I would find the light waiting to welcome me home.

I drew tremendous strength and a sense of unshakable peace each time I remembered the experience, piece by piece. Even as I put each piece in place I never lost my sense of the whole sensation.

It was the most profound experience of my life. I shared it with no one. I just kept remembering the light and took much comfort in the memory.

I finally left the hospital in late January after more than a month of intensive care.

Kenny

We were placed on AZT therapy. AZT had just been approved by the Food and Drug Administration (FDA) because it appeared to slow the virus' progress. We were told AZT might have some serious side effects, including intense nausea and vomiting.

Barbra

After returning home I felt agitated and cranky. Once again all I wanted to do was sleep. I had quit my job while hospitalized and did not go out and look for another. The sight and smell of food still made me sick to my stomach.

Kenny and I were still not talking and I did not share my experience with the light with Kenny. The person I had come back to help was not yet willing to be helped. This made me feel frustrated and crabby. But I knew the time would come and things would work out as they should.

Kenny

Shortly after we were diagnosed we began going to group meetings run by the Bay County Health Department for HIV patients. While most members of this group are gay, Barbra and I got along well with them. After all, we shared a similar disease.

During one of these meetings we began talking with another AIDS patient who, like Barbra, had a serious problem with weight loss and protracted nausea and vomiting. He told us smoking marijuana helped to reduce the nausea and control the vomiting. He also said marijuana would make us want to eat.

Barbra

Kenny and I spoke to this man in the parking lot for many hours after our meeting was over. He was a very nice man and seemed to genuinely want to help us. Both Kenny and I had heard cancer patients often smoke marijuana to control the debilitating side effects of anti-cancer drugs. But we had never considered smoking marijuana to help with our AIDS.

The man gently encouraged us to smoke some marijuana. He said it only took a few puffs to make the nausea go away. I wanted to believe him, but couldn't.

My doctors had already prescribed more than a half dozen anti-nausea drugs in an effort to control my nausea and vomiting and stop my drastic weight loss. None of these prescription drugs worked. I simply could not tolerate the sight or smell or taste of food. If all these so-called "miracle drugs" prescribed by my doctors failed to work I didn't see how smoking an illegal weed like marijuana was going to make me feel any better.

Kenny

I had smoked marijuana occasionally during my youth, but I did not find marijuana all that interesting. If given a choice I preferred a good cold beer. Besides, I respect the law and do not like doing anything illegal. This is probably because of my father's military and law enforcement background. He is still an active U.S. Customs agent.

The man, however, insisted marijuana might help. And he gave me a marijuana cigarette. He told me to smoke it after I got home and said I'd notice the difference right away.

Barbra was extremely skeptical. The doctors had prescribed a number of powerful anti-nausea drugs in an effort to control her vomiting and weight loss. But nothing the doctors prescribed seemed to help. She was constantly sick to her stomach and, despite the prescribed drugs, was literally fading away.

Barbra

The man told us he too had been skeptical, he too had tried all the prescription drugs. When we finally said good-night he gave us some marijuana to take with us. He told us we should use it whenever we felt sick to our stomachs. Kenny and I were always sick to our stomachs. On the drive home we briefly discussed the idea of smoking marijuana. I bluntly told Kenny I was not about to smoke marijuana because I didn't want to become a drug addict. I told him if he wanted to smoke marijuana it was his life.

Kenny had smoked marijuana while growing up. I had never smoked marijuana or done anything illegal. And, after my bout with pneumonia I had stopped smoking tobacco. I could not imagine putting any more smoke into my lungs. Gasping for air is a horrible experience. It teaches you to enjoy breathing.

When we got home Kenny thought about smoking. It was nearly midnight when he came to me and said he was going to try the marijuana we had been given. We went into the living room and I watched as Kenny lit the cigarette.

Kenny

I took a few puffs from the cigarette and almost immediately something changed. My body seemed to relax. My sore joints seemed less stiff. Then I realized my nausea—that just-about-to-be-sick feeling that had been with me for months—had suddenly vanished.

I was astonished. I took just a few more puffs and continued to feel better and better. It was amazing. I started telling Barbra about how different I felt. She began asking me lots of questions. Within 10 minutes were we talking together, and we were talking about our disease—AIDS. It was like a dam broke. For the first time since the doctor told us we might be infected we were having a normal conversation.

I told Barbra I was sorry, that it was my fault she was infected, that she should never have married me. And she told me that being sick was no one's fault, that she understood how bad I must feel, and that it was time for us to make the best of what was happening to us.

It was our first honest talk in years. And it brought us closer together.

About an hour after I smoked marijuana I found myself in the kitchen looking for something, anything to eat. I was literally starving and marijuana had suddenly given me back my appetite. I ate nearly anything and everything in sight. It was just so wonderful to eat. Barbra watched me eat and we kept talking. For the first time in months we made jokes and laughed together.

When we went to bed Barbra tried to sleep but I kept talking.

Barbra

Kenny smoked a small amount of marijuana. A short time (10-15 minutes) later he said he felt better. I remained skeptical. I remember thinking maybe Kenny just thought he felt better.

Kenny started to talk. It had been so long since we had sat together and talked. For the first time we talked about AIDS. Kenny told me how sorry he was I had gotten sick. How he felt my sickness was his fault — if he did not have hemophilia we would not have AIDS. For the first time Kenny confronted the guilt, grief, and pain we had both been feeling for nearly two years — ever since the doctor first told us about the tainted blood.

It was like walking into sunlight. The pent-up anguish and dark emotions, our unspoken fears and deepest concerns came rushing out.

It allowed me, for the first time, to tell Kenny I understood his pain and guilt. I explained AIDS is just a part of life. Would he be guilty if, because we lived together, I got a cold? For the first time in a long time we were together. And for the first time we were confronting our problems instead of running away from them.

We actually laughed. That may not seem like anything special. But being able to laugh together made a tremendous difference at that moment to our lives. It had been a long time since we'd smiled at one another. We cried together.

About an hour after Kenny smoked the marijuana he raided the kitchen. I watched amused and amazed as my husband ate. It was a wonderful thing to see. To me it was nearly impossible to believe. Kenny consumed every kind of food he could find. Watching him stuff food into his mouth made me joyful and envious, and caused me to remember my own, unrelieved nausea. I began to think about smoking marijuana. Maybe it could help.

Kenny

After Barbra fell asleep, I did a lot of thinking. I realized my life had been out of control. I was so scared, guilty and hurt by all that was happening to me that I wasn't enjoying the life I had left. Then I fell into a deep, wonderful sleep.

Barbra

The next day, while Kenny was at work, I thought about the night before. Kenny seemed like his old self. We had gotten along so well, unburdened our souls of so much hurt and confusion. And he really had eaten a lot of food. If smoking just a small amount of marijuana could do all that I decided it was worth trying.

When Kenny got home he came straight into the house to smoke the rest of the marijuana we had been given. He asked me if I wanted to join him. My heart racing, I said "yes."

Within seconds of taking my first puff I felt the tightness in my stomach ease. A few more puffs and my whole body unclenched. Within 15 minutes the gnawing nausea in the pit of my stomach was gone. Gone! Kenny and I talked about these things as they happened, sharing the experience, looking for clues.

All my life I have been told marijuana is a dangerous drug. I didn't see any danger. What I did notice was a complete change in my sense of things. My constant nausea was gone. That alone was astonishing. The doctors had given me all sorts of prescription anti-nausea drugs, but they hadn't worked. Just a few puffs of a marijuana cigarette, however, made my nausea vanish. It was like a miracle.

Kenny

We sat down together and smoked the rest of the marijuana cigarette. Then we settled in for another long evening of talking, laughing, and eating. It was great to see my wife smiling and eating again.

Barbra

Kenny and I talked about so many things. Then, like Kenny the night before, I became truly hungry. I was famished—literally starving. And I was overwhelmed by a desire to eat. I had not eaten a complete meal in months, had not been able to even think of food without gagging for three months. Now, suddenly, I could not eat enough food fast enough.

I felt as if my body had been released from prison. The more I ate the better I felt. I became giddy with delight. I thought about how good life is and, suddenly, my illness came into perspective. For the first time I felt I was coping with my disease.

Marijuana did not make AIDS any less frightening. But I came to realize people die everyday from a host of terrible diseases and unexpected accidents. AIDS is simply another terrible disease, an accident in my life. It is difficult to explain how important this realization is to me. In a way it is the realization of my near-death experience brought into my daily life.

Marijuana allowed me to separate the really important from the merely frightening. After smoking marijuana the horrible sense of chaos, of being out of control, disappeared like a phantom. In its place came a calm assurance. Sure I had AIDS—so do lots of other people. To use an old cliche, instead of gripping because life handed me a lemon I was suddenly making lemonade. This shift in attitude—in my way of dealing with AIDS—made a world of difference.

After an orgy of eating, talking, laughing, and reflecting, Kenny and I went to bed and, for the first night in months, I got a restful night's sleep.

Kenny

After that experience our lives returned to normal. I'd get up in the morning and go off to work. Barbra would stay home, clean the trailer, play with our pets. Then she would fix dinner. I'd come home, we would sit down and smoke a marijuana cigarette together, then we'd eat dinner and discuss our day.

Barbra

After that night Kenny and I vowed we would smoke marijuana as part of our medical treatment. We knew it was illegal. But we decided our immediate medical needs were a lot more important. Without marijuana we would simply starve to death. We did not think it was "criminal" for us to eat and stay healthy.

Kenny

At first we got marijuana from our friend in the AIDS group. He grew his own marijuana and it was excellent. We only needed to smoke a couple of puffs to get relief. Then he moved away. So we began asking other people if they could find us marijuana. But we hardly told anyone we were HIV+ or that Barbra had AIDS. We pretended to be social smokers. Eventually, through a friend or a friend of a friend we managed to purchase a small amount of marijuana.

It was hard to find and afford enough marijuana to meet our medical needs. Sometimes we could afford marijuana, but could not find any to buy. When we didn't smoke marijuana we quickly relapsed, started feeling sick, and would be unable to eat.

In an effort to make sure Barbra and I had the marijuana we needed I decided to grow two small plants. Then, when we couldn't find marijuana to buy, we'd at least have enough to smoke to tide us over until we could find more.

Barbra

I did not tell my doctors. We didn't know how they might react and we were afraid they might turn us in to the police. Kenny did, however, at one point ask his doctor about marijuana, and if there was anything like a legal "pot pill" that he could prescribe. The doctor told Kenny a kind of "pot pill" existed, but that it could only be prescribed to cancer patients. Since we didn't have cancer he said he could not provide it to us. The doctor also said the pill was expensive and did not seem to work well. It seems the doctor did not have a very high opinion of the synthetic marijuana pill.

Kenny

Whenever I brought the subject of marijuana up to my doctor, however, he'd just tell me it was illegal. The doctor indicated we were not the only patients smoking marijuana and it was not the first time he'd heard of marijuana being used to control nausea and vomiting. It seemed like a crazy catch-22.

But we managed and things seemed to be going well. We stayed out of the hospital and stayed well. I continued working as a security alarm installer.

Barbra

For the next year things went very well. I was hospitalized for a week in early-April 1989 when my pneumonia tried to come back, and I continued to have a problem with yeast infections. But for nearly a year Kenny and I stayed healthy, ate fairly well, and maintained our weight.

Prior to smoking marijuana my days were deadly dull. I would get up in the morning, walk into the bathroom and throw-up, walk into the living room, lie down on the sofa and wallow in depression. I would stay on that sofa all day, except for frequent trips to the bathroom to throw-up. I would not have anything to eat. Occasionally, I might fall into a fitful sleep.

I stopped making dinner because the look and smell of food made me gag. Besides, neither Kenny nor I could eat dinner once it was cooked. It got to the point Kenny, if he ate anything at all, picked up something on his way home from work and ate it in the car. That way I did not have to smell food in the house.

Marijuana changed this routine dramatically. In the morning Kenny would make me a small marijuana cigarette before he left for work. I would get up, walk to the living room, smoke a few puffs then get on with my day. When lunchtime came I would eat lunch. I might take a short nap in the afternoon. When it came time to fix dinner I would smoke a few more puffs, and make dinner. Kenny would come home. We would sit down together and we would eat. Just like old times.

Relieved of my constant nausea I was also relieved of my sense of foreboding. My chronic depression disappeared. I wanted to do things, get out of the house, play with my pets, enjoy the life left me. My energy slowly returned and I began to slowly gain weight.

In every sense of the word, marijuana made a critical difference in my medical care. We were not throwing-up. We were eating well and our weight was coming back. Kenny, despite his low T-cell count, continued working and bringing home a paycheck. Our mood was good.

Because we were eating well, we were able to continue taking AZT, the only drug known to help retard the HIV virus. Many patients, unable to tolerate the intense nausea and vomiting of AIDS and AZT therapy, are forced to quit AZT. Unable to tolerate treatment, their disease becomes progressive and they rapidly fall prey to opportunistic infections.

Marijuana helped us avoid this dangerous trap. Of course, there were times when we could not buy marijuana. Either we could not afford it or we could not locate someone to buy it from. The effects of being without marijuana were equally dramatic in the wrong direction. We would quickly begin to get nauseated, our appetites would decrease, I would end up back on the sofa, depressed, worried, throwing-up. Then we would get a small amount of marijuana and our appetites and spirits would quickly revive.

In an effort to avoid this problem, Kenny decided to grow two marijuana plants. He reasoned two small plants would be enough to get us through the hard times when we simply could not find or afford marijuana to meet our medical needs.

I was apprehensive about growing marijuana. But not nearly as apprehensive as I was about being without any marijuana and suffering the consequences.

We went on like this for a year. Our health was stable, our spirits good. We stayed out of the hospital and with each other. Odd as this may seem, we were generally happy. I thank God for each day I am alive and try to make the best of each day.

Kenny

Then, on the evening of March 29, 1990, our home was surrounded by 8 to 10 armed men. Before I could go to the door they smashed it in with a battering ram. They aimed their guns at me and one pointed his pistol directly at Barbra's head. They ordered us around and began tearing our home apart. We had been invaded by the Bay County Narcotics Task Force.

The vice agents conducted a long search and tore our trailer apart. Then they brought the evidence into our living room. They had found my two small marijuana plants. The largest was about 10 inches tall; the other was only 4 inches tall. Vice agents examined my infusion syringes and accused me of being a heroin addict. I explained I suffered from hemophilia.

Barbra and I were handcuffed and taken to the Task Force headquarters, then to the Bay County jail where our fingerprints and mug shots were taken. Then we were booked.

Before being taken to jail the narcotics officers interrogated me and my wife. They demanded I give them the names and addresses of all the people to whom I sold marijuana. I have never sold marijuana to anyone. They told me they were going to put me in jail for years unless I gave them the names of my "contacts." I did not have any contacts, just a few people willing to help Barbra and me find the marijuana we medically needed.

Barbra

The vice agents said Kenny and I were in serious trouble—on our way to prison for a long, long time. The men were gruff and threatening. They demanded the names and addresses of all the people to whom we sold marijuana. They acted as if Kenny and I were major drug traffickers. We never sold any marijuana. We needed it too badly to sell it to others.

Then we were taken to jail, fingerprinted, photographed, strip-searched, and put into cells. We had heard frightening stories of how AIDS patients were abused in prisons. But, when the guard asked me about any diseases I might have I blurted out I had tuberculosis (TB) and was HIV+. She did not seem to understand what I was saying. I certainly did not repeat it.

I was put in a cold, filthy cell with one other women. It was freezing and I was a still in a state of shock. Just hours before I had been fixing dinner for Kenny. Now, I was suddenly behind bars, being treated like a major criminal.

I asked one of the guards for a blanket. I didn't get one. After freezing in that cold cell for hours I was transferred to the Bay County Jail Annex, and placed in another dirty cell.

I barely slept that night. I kept wondering if Kenny was alright. I also wondered what would become of us. I have never been in trouble with the law and did not have the first idea what to do. I did not know anything about bail or how to get out.

After making dozens of phone calls, Kenny and I were finally released on bail at around 6:00 p.m. the next evening. It was one of the most bewildering experiences I have ever had. One result of the arrest: Kenny was fired from his job as a security alarm installer.

Kenny

When we got home neither of us could eat—we were nauseated and there was no marijuana. We talked about what had happened to us and the more we talked the madder we got. How could the police arrest us for using a drug that helped keep us alive? We decided that if there was any way to fight being called "criminals" we were ready to do so, even if this meant everyone in Bay County would find out we had AIDS. We were not going to put up with it anymore.

That weekend I went out and purchased a drug magazine called *High Times*. I hoped I could find help by reading the magazine. I found a lot more than I'd been looking for.

To my complete surprise I ran across an article about a Texas man who had just become the first AIDS patient to receive FDA permission to legally smoke marijuana to help control the nausea and vomiting associated with his disease. The article was written by Robert Randall. It contained a phone number that patients in need of help could call.

Barbra

Kenny called the number and within an hour Mr. Robert Randall phoned us back and asked how he could help. Kenny explained our situation. Mr. Randall explained we could obtain legal marijuana from the federal government if our doctors would apply on our behalf.

We quickly discovered our local doctors were unwilling to apply to get us legal access to marijuana. It was not that they doubted marijuana helped us deal with nausea and vomiting. They knew better than that. Put simply, our local doctors were too afraid to help us. After all, Kenny and I are considered "drug criminals" by the police. The local doctors do not want to cross the Bay County Narcotics Task Force. Who would?

Kenny

We phoned Mr. Randall and told him the bad news. He told us he would try to locate a doctor in North Florida who specialized in treating hemophilia and AIDS. He expressed concern about the quality of medical care we had received in Bay County. He also said he would look for a good criminal lawyer to represent us in court.

It sounded real good, but I thought he was pulling my leg. We had no money. How could we possibly afford an expensive criminal lawyer? After our local doctors refused to help us I doubted Mr. Randall would be able to find a doctor willing to assist us. In our experience, doctors seemed terrified whenever they dealt with us.

Barbra

Mr. Randall arranged for us to meet a doctor in Pensacola. The doctor specialized in AIDS treatments. I was especially pleased to learn our new doctor, Thomas Sonnenberg, also specialized in hematology (the study of blood) and knew a great deal about hemophilia. Mr. Randall apologized the doctor was so far away from Bay County (about 120 miles).

We were delighted that a doctor who knew something about AIDS was willing to see us. We made an appointment and saw the doctor. It was certainly worth the trip. For the first time since Kenny and I got AIDS we met a doctor who did not seem to be afraid of us.

Our new doctor asked each of us lots of very detailed questions about our illness. He took time to answer our simplest questions. He noticed I had a very bad yeast infection—an infection I'd had for nearly two years. After consulting with a local pharmacist the doctor prescribed a drug my own doctors had never tried. Four days later my yeast infection was gone.

After reviewing our case, Dr. Sonnenberg agreed to work with Mr. Randall to help us apply to get legal access to U.S. government-grown marijuana. Dr. Sonnenberg told us a large number of patients with cancer and AIDS smoke marijuana to reduce nausea and vomiting. Through Mr. Randall, Dr. Sonnenberg could learn how to apply for legal marijuana.

Doctor Sonnenberg's knowledge of hemophilia greatly eased my mind. Kenny needs special medical attention and Dr. Sonnenberg seemed very attuned to his needs. Dr. Sonnenberg promised to explore ways to get Kenny supplies of Factor VIII he could take home so he can promptly infuse himself when necessary.

Dr. Sonnenberg also has expressed concern about my own bleeding problem. For many months I have had an almost uninterrupted kind of menstrual bleeding. Dr. Sonnenberg prescribed a new medicine in an effort to control this bleeding. Initially, the new drug worked, and my bleeding stopped.

Within several weeks, however, my bleeding recurred. Finally, it became so bad I contacted Dr. Sonnenberg. He asked me to come in for a check up that afternoon and, after doing some basic blood work, he placed me in a hospital in Pensacola.

I remained in the hospital over the weekend and a biopsy was taken from my uterus. Clearly, the doctors are concerned that my constant bleeding suggests I may be developing an AIDS-related cancer.

Dr. Sonnenberg's knowledge of cancer, AIDS, and hematology has been a great benefit to Kenny and me. My own gynecologist in Bay County was aware of my bleeding problem, but did nothing to stop it. While my pap smears were ominous, my local doctor showed almost no concern. Indeed, at one point my own doctor told me I should look elsewhere for medical care.

Kenny

Mr. Randall then arranged for us to be represented by one of the best criminal defense lawyers in Northern Florida, Mr. John Daniel. Mr. Randall told us that Mr. Daniel came highly recommended. He encouraged us to make an appointment to see Mr. Daniel as soon as possible. We learned Mr. Daniel had agreed to represent us without charge. But Mr. Randall said if we were not comfortable with Mr. Daniel he would arrange for us to meet with another attorney.

Our meeting with Mr. Daniel went extremely well. He was clearly interested in our case. He explained he was working for us, but that Mr. Randall and others in Washington were providing him with lots of helpful background information. He told us not to worry. We felt we were in very good hands.

Barbra

Since our arrest I have discovered that a lot of AIDS patients, and people with cancer, glaucoma, multiple sclerosis, and other crippling diseases, medically smoke marijuana for relief. Doctors and patients discuss marijuana's medical use all the time. Yet, only a handful of Americans have the legal right to smoke marijuana. Meanwhile, tens of thousands of other patients, like Kenny and me, are forced to get the marijuana we medically need off the streets.

This is outrageous. Doctors who can prescribe toxic anti-cancer drugs, addictive morphine, and powerful AZT treatments are legally prohibited from prescribing marijuana! Marijuana is one of the few drugs I have been given that has done me no harm and made it possible for me to live with AIDS. This medically effective plant is illegal while pharmacies filled with expensive, extremely dangerous, and usually ineffective drugs are handed out like candy. This is more than outrageous—it's crazy.

Kenny

For the "crime" of growing two small marijuana plants we are charged with three major felonies: 1) cultivation of marijuana with intent to distribute, 2) possession of a Schedule I substance, and 3) possession of drug paraphernalia.

We intend to raise a legal defense of "medical necessity" and we intend to win. Barbra and I are done being scared. We realize there are thousands of other AIDS and cancer patients who could benefit from marijuana's anti-nausea and appetite stimulating effects. We believe it is wrong for the government to ignore our legitimate medical needs or the medical needs of these other patients.

Barbra

Kenny and I decided there would be no plea bargaining. It is true we grew two small marijuana plants. But I am not a criminal and I am not going to allow anyone to treat me like a criminal. And I am not going to stand by and let policemen take away the one drug that helps me cope with AIDS. We made it very clear to Mr. Daniel we did not want to strike a deal. We wanted to fight the charges.

We plan to fight—and fight hard. And I know we are going to win. I am very confident of this. And I know because we have been arrested, and because there is going to be a trial that thousands of other patients with AIDS all around the United States are going to know — many for the first time—that marijuana can help them, too.

Kenny

We hope our trial helps other patients learn about marijuana's medical use. Whether legal or illegal, marijuana works. That is what is important when you are desperately ill. I sincerely believe Barbra would have died without marijuana's appetite stimulating properties. And I believe without marijuana my own condition would have progressed to full-blown AIDS.

Barbra and I have no illusions. We realize AIDS remains a deadly disease. And we also realize we are asking people to confront and overcome their fears — of AIDS and of marijuana — and to understand that we are seriously ill patients, not criminals.

The only crime I see is the government prohibition against the medical use of a drug that has such clear and obvious medical benefits.

Barbra

A year ago, even two months ago, I lived in great fear. I was afraid of being sick. I was afraid our friends and neighbors would find out we have AIDS. But I know I am right and I am not afraid of anybody anymore. And if all the trauma of our being arrested ends up helping one other AIDS patient sit down and eat a decent meal I will leave this world feeling I helped someone in need of help. In the end that's what living is all about.

✦ ✦ ✦ ✦

In June 1990, Kenny and Barbra's physician applied to the FDA for permission to legally prescribe marijuana to help control their AZT-induced nausea, vomiting, and weight loss.

In July 1990, Kenny and Barbra went on trial. The local court refused to heed the testimony of two medical experts and dismissed the Jenks' claim of "medical necessity." In August 1990, the court found them guilty of three felony counts. Kenny and Barbra were sentenced to: 1) serve one year of unsupervised probation, 2) do 500 hours of "community service," which the judge defined as "loving and caring for one another," and 3) withheld adjudication. In effect, if Kenny and Barbra stayed out of trouble for one year the record in their case would be voided.

In October 1990, Kenny and Barbra Jenks asked Florida Governor Bob Martinez for a pardon. Martinez lost the November 1990 election and left office before hearing their pardon request.

In December 1990, the FDA, after more than six months of delays, approved their physician's request for compassionate IND access to medicinal supplies of marijuana. The Drug Enforcement Administration (DEA), however, refused to authorize their shipment. Finally, on February 19, 1991, eight full months after their doctor filed his initial IND application, Barbra and Kenny Jenks became the third and fourth AIDS patients in the United States to legally obtain federal supplies of medicinal marijuana under the FDA's cumbersome compassionate IND procedures.

On February 28, 1991, Mr. and Mrs. Jenks joined Robert Randall and Chicago financier Richard J. Dennis in Chicago to announce the formation of the MARS project.

MARS—the Marijuana·AIDS Research Service—is designed to empower HIV+ people and their physicians in applying to FDA for Compassionate IND access to government supplies of medicinal marijuana. (See page 115).

Since its inception MARS has received a constant stream of requests from HIV+ people for assistance. At this writing more than 400 MARS packets have been sent to HIV+ patients. Hundreds of MARS-based compassionate IND applications have been copied by local AIDS support groups around the United States and provided to HIV+ people.

On April 17, 1991, the Florida Court of Appeals reversed the lower court verdict and ruled that Kenny and Barbra Jenks were not guilty of marijuana possession by reason of "medical necessity." The decision marked the first time a U.S. Court has declared marijuana to be a drug of "medical necessity" in the treatment of HIV infection.

The State of Florida attempted to overturn the Court of Appeals verdict by appealing to the Florida Supreme Court but on October 8, 1991, the Court refused to hear the case. The Jenks gratefully acknowledged the Court's action. "We didn't want to die as convicted felons," said Kenny Jenks.

Mr. and Mrs. Jenks remain active and outspoken defenders of marijuana's medical availability to HIV+ individuals. In late 1991, they were featured on a segment of the CBS News program 60 Minutes. In November 1991, the Drug Policy Foundation, a Washington-based drug policy think-tank, awarded Mr. and Mrs. Jenks the Robert C. Randall Citizen Achievement Award with an accompanying $10,000 cash award, in recognition of their efforts on behalf of other seriously ill Americans.

Chapter Four

DANNY

It's just been terribly frustrating dealing with the government on this issue and fighting the bureaucratic maze. They almost make it so complicated that is sets up people to fail.

Danny, Second person with AIDS
to gain legal, medical
access to marijuana.
October 1990

The Jenks were not the only people with AIDS (PWAs) who read about Steve's success in acquiring legal access to marijuana. Throughout the first half of 1990, several PWAs and people with HIV infection called the Alliance for Cannabis Therapeutics (ACT) for information on how they could acquire marijuana legally. The compassionate IND process was explained to each one. In some cases, like the Jenks, assistance was located. Others tried to convince their doctors to help but the doctors refused. In at least one instance a compassionate IND was prepared but the patient became too weak to pursue legal access and died during the summer months. Others simply listened and made the determination that the compassionate IND was too much of a hassle. Life was too short for these PWAs to spend precious time rankling with federal agencies. Street marijuana was expensive, scarce, and illegal, but in the long run, it was easier.

In May 1990, the Alliance received a call from a Northern Virginia man who had read about Steve's case. This individual, a gay white male who worked as a registered psychiatric nurse in a Washington area hospital, had discovered that marijuana helped maintain his weight and decreased the nausea caused by AZT. Initially he had refused to believe that marijuana was helping him. This is not uncommon with people who use marijuana medically. Over time, however, it became apparent that marijuana was a critical element in his care. He had become increasingly anxious about using the drug illegally and finally decided to call. The compassionate IND process was explained and the man was encouraged to discuss the matter with his doctor. Several days later the man called back and said his doctor was willing to help.

Throughout the next several months the Alliance worked with this man to prepare and submit the IND. The following news accounts of the case first appeared in *The Blade*, Washington, D.C.'s gay newspaper. For reasons relating to his work and family, the man chose to remain anonymous and is known only as *Danny*. In addition to the following articles, Danny's case was reported in the popular press and he appeared, in shadow, on a local newscast.

Danny was the second HIV+ individual to gain legal access to marijuana. As this book goes to press, Danny reports his health is generally good and credits marijuana with making a "substantial difference" in his medical therapy. He has high praise for his doctor who "was compassionate enough to apply in the first place and courageous enough to stay the course after all these federal agencies started to hassle him."

Should other individuals with AIDS apply for legal access to marijuana? "If it helps them, they should," says Danny. "But you have to be stubborn and patient—a difficult combination of emotions. Be prepared for anything. And forget common sense—if logic prevailed you could walk into your pharmacy and get marijuana, the same as any other drug. The federal government doesn't want people to have medical marijuana and there is very little compassion in the compassionate IND."

VIRGINIA PWA BATTLES TO GET MARIJUANA TO EASE SYMPTOMS[*]

by Nick Bartolomeo

A Northern Virginia man with AIDS has been caught in the crossfire of the war on drugs.

The man, who is Gay but agreed to be interviewed for this article only on the condition that he not be identified, is a registered nurse with a D.C. metropolitan area health care facility. On June 18, he received permission from the Food and Drug Administration to obtain marijuana legally for treatment of AIDS-related nausea, vomiting, and weight loss. But, more than four months later, the man has yet to obtain his first legal marijuana cigarette.

The problem, he said, lies with the Drug Enforcement Agency. DEA's role in the unwieldy process is to ensure that a person's physician is legitimate and that his pharmacy is secure enough to handle the substance. But according to the Northern Virginia man, his physician has not yet been contacted by the agency, and DEA employees seemed less than sympathetic to his plight.

"It's just been terribly frustrating dealing with the government on this issue and fighting the bureaucratic maze," said the man. "They almost make it so complicated that it sets up people" to fail. The man said that when he called a Washington DEA official Oct. 16 to check on the agency's progress, he was told that the FDA had not yet notified the agency that his request for legal marijuana was approved. But when he contacted FDA the same day, he said, he was told that DEA was notified of the approval several weeks earlier.

---

[*]   Originally published in *The Washington Blade*, October 26, 1990. Reprinted with permission.

The man said he then called DEA the following day, and the same DEA official told him that
the agency had indeed received approval over the
telephone from FDA. But, said the man, the DEA
still refused to accept the approval and
demanded that the FDA put the authorization in
writing.

"It brings out a lot of anger at the government
for being so inefficient," said the Gay man. "It's
really anxiety provoking, and it shouldn't have to
be that way."

DEA Public Affairs Spokesperson Joe Keefe
would not comment on specifics in the case. An
FDA spokesperson did not respond to a reporter's
question by *Blade* deadline.

Robert Randall, president of the Alliance for
Cannabis Therapeutics, a nonprofit D.C. organization working to legalize the medicinal use [of]
marijuana, said DEA's behavior comes as no
surprise.

"Sadly, it's the same old routine," said Randall. "DEA is dealing in dogma in fighting a war
on drugs, and it wants to fight that war in black
and white. It won't admit that marijuana is a
plant that has good and bad uses."

Randall said that DEA has ignored a 1988
ruling by its own chief administrative law judge
that marijuana should be made available by
prescription for medicinal purposes. DEA's
stance, said Randall, was instrumental in delay-
ing marijuana treatment for a Texas man who
late last year became the first person with AIDS
to legally receive marijuana.

In that case, Randall said, the DEA
"stonewalled" the Texas man's attempt to get the
drug after receiving FDA approval, and, according
to San Antonio AIDS Foundation Director Robert
Edwards, reportedly told its San Antonio office
"not to be in a rush about it."

The DEA authorized the marijuana shipment
Jan. 16. Steve died Feb. 2.

In 1976, Randall became the first person to
obtain marijuana legally for a medical ailment
under the Compassionate Investigational New
Drug (IND) program, which he helped originate.

The Compassionate IND program was the forerunner of the Treatment IND program, under which the AIDS therapy drugs AZT and ddi were released outside clinical trials to people with AIDS.

The Northern Virginia man with AIDS said that he came to Randall for help in procuring marijuana after Marinol, a prescription drug containing marijuana's active ingredient, THC, failed to help him.

"I was miserable," said the Northern Virginia man, who was also experiencing side effects from AZT. "Just brushing my teeth would initiate gagging and then vomiting, and the vomiting would not seem to stop."

After smoking marijuana which he had obtained illegally, he said, his nausea and the muscles spasms subsided.

"I got very hungry after I smoked," said the Gay man. "Being able to eat, I have really been able to gain back some of the lost weight."

The man said he decided to try to obtain marijuana legally because street access had "dried up" and he was concerned about risking arrest.

"I also hoped that, in some way, I could make it easier for other persons with AIDS down the road to get marijuana for their symptoms," said the man.

The Northern Virginia man said he also met Monday with an aide to Sen. John Warner (R-Va.), whom he said told him that the Senator's office "would try to speed things along" at DEA "if there has been a hold up." Warner Staff Assistant Sean Mullen would not confirm that such a meeting had taken place, but noted that Warner "makes every effort to help constituents facing difficulties with a federal agency."

Randall indicated that the Northern Virginia man's case would prove to be important for people with AIDS trying to procure the drug legally in the future.

"Each time one person goes through" the procurement process," said Randall, "it will make

it easier for others to follow. I expect thousands,
if not tens of thousands, of AIDS patients to follow."

✛ ✛ ✛ ✛

DEA APPROVES MARIJUANA
FOR VIRGINIA PWA*

by Nick Bartolomeo

The U.S. Drug Enforcement Administration
last week approved a request by a Gay Northern
Virginia man to receive marijuana for use in treating the side effects of AIDS. The event marked
only the second time that a person with AIDS has
legally received the drug.

"Thanks to the marijuana, I've been able to
eat," said the 34-year old Gay man, who spoke
only on the condition that he not be identified. "I
feel that a big source of stress in my life has been
eliminated, at least for the time being.

The Gay man, a health care professional, had
petitioned the government last June for permission to receive marijuana under a program which
releases the highly-controlled drug for medicinal
use. According to the Gay man, marijuana al-
leviated his AIDS-related nausea and lack of appetite.

The Gay man said that the FDA approved his
request within two weeks but that it was stalled
for five months by DEA. The DEA must verify the
legitimacy of the petitioner's physician, who acts
as a coordinator and a researcher in the process,
and confirm that the pharmacy receiving the
drug is secure. The marijuana itself is shipped by
yet another federal agency, the National Institute
of Drug Abuse.

---

* Originally published in *The Washington Blade*, November 30, 1990.
Reprinted with permission.

However, DEA spokesperson Bill Ruzzamenti said that the agency received the necessary paperwork from the Gay man's physician only on Sept. 11. Ruzzamenti said that the process usually takes 30 to 90 days, and the request for the Gay man was approved on Nov. 19.

Alliance for Cannabis Therapeutics President Robert Randall, who assisted the Gay man in his request to the government, said that the delay was the result of inherent complications in the system and should lessen when more AIDS patients request the drug.

"The more often the system deals with this, the quicker it will respond," said Randall, whose organization is lobbying for reform in marijuana medicinal use laws. "This is a therapy that works, and AIDS patients have every right to get it."

DEA spokesperson Bill Ruzzamenti said that the marijuana medicinal use process "is in place" and that the Administration has "no plans" to change it to accommodate the time-sensitive requests by people with AIDS, whose health can often deteriorate quickly.

The Gay man said that people with AIDS wishing to obtain the drug should make certain to have a "dedicated physician."

"That's what it takes, someone who is going to stick it out," said the Gay man. "It's not an easy thing to do."

The first person with AIDS to receive marijuana was a Texas man identified in news reports only as "Steve." In that case, marijuana advocates and Gay activists alleged that DEA had thwarted the procurement process to deny Steve the drug, even though he had obtained FDA approval. On Jan. 16, 1990, DEA authorized Steve's request. He died a few weeks later.

Chapter Five

A DOCTOR'S PERSPECTIVE

*The patients in my office, in my experience, are not
smoking to get high, to get euphoric, to freak out, to
jump from roof to roof. They're smoking marijuana to
get relief of suffering, which is really what medical oncology is about.*

Ivan Silverberg, M.D.
December 1987

In late 1987, as part of court-ordered public hearings on
marijuana's medical utility, Administrative Law Judge Francis Young
of the Drug Enforcement Administration (DEA) heard testimony in
San Francisco, California. Among the witnesses was Dr. Ivan Silverberg, an oncologist with offices near San Francisco's Castro district.
He is on staff at the University of California at San Francisco Hospital
and is an associate professor of Clinical Oncology and Radiology at
the University of California at San Francisco. During his testimony,
Dr. Silverberg discussed how his clientele has changed in recent years
from older patients with cancer to young men with AIDS.

The use of marijuana by AIDS patients is similar to that of cancer
patients. For both afflictions marijuana provides relief from
chemotherapeutically induced nausea and vomiting. It also provides
appetite stimulation, which allows the patient to retain body weight
and better fight other opportunistic ailments.

When Ivan Silverberg testified in December 1987, Steve L. was living
through his fifth month with full-blown AIDS. Steve had already
realized that marijuana was helping him and he was beginning to
wonder how he could legally obtain the marijuana he medically
needed. Barbra and Kenny Jenks had just learned Kenny received an
HIV+ transfusion. They were living a private nightmare of denial, fear,
and panic.

For Ivan Silverberg the use of marijuana by AIDS patients was nothing unusual. As a practicing oncologist he had been aware of marijuana's medical utility for many years and he encouraged his patients to do whatever they could to relieve the nausea and vomiting.

The following exchange is the only mention of marijuana's use by AIDS patients during the DEA hearings. Dr. Silverberg was questioned by Frank Stilwell, attorney for the Alliance for Cannabis Therapeutics.

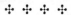

Q. Just how bad is this vomiting?

A. It varies. Currently, if I were to take my commonest cancer, which is AIDS-related lymphosarcoma, a disease in a non-cured situation has a median survival of six months or less, I would think that 90 to 95% of my patients will vomit during their three-week course, repetitively.

Most of them by the third or fourth week will start vomiting. Most of them, I tell them by the eighth or ninth week they're going to hate me and most of them do.

Q. What sort of impact does that vomiting pattern have upon their life, the patient's life?

A. It's hard to answer that one realistically.

It's a terrifying experience. It's terrifying to go home, to be alone, to be 30 years old, to be dying of a malignancy, and to be throwing up. It's terrifying to loose weight because you can't hold food down. It's devastating to my patients.

Q. Does marijuana improve the quality of life?

A. In my office, in my experience, yes. It decreases dramatically the incidence of vomiting in patient after patient after patient. And I can give you stories; I unfortunately cannot get patient permission to use names, but over and over again it decreases vomiting and it improves appetite.

Q. *Doctor, do you think the American Medical Association (AMA) should be the standard for determining what accepted medical use is in the United States?*

A. Not hardly.

Q. *Why?*

A. They're a legal organization. I think it would be the same as any organization of any professional group of people trying to say how an office should be run.

I don't think that the American Medical Association has adequate representation, if for no other reason, on their executive and decision making bodies of people who are dealing with drugs that cause nausea and vomiting.

I think that if you go through the AMA presidents over the last 10 or 15 years, I'm sure you won't find a medical oncologist among them. I don't think you'll find one on the board.

Lawrence P. White, who is running for the California Medical Association presidency is the first medical oncologist in the state of California, to my knowledge, to be in such a position.

So, it's representation and decision making on medical grounds by internists, cardiologists, gastroenterologists, general practitioners, people of this sort not by medical oncologists who are there emptying the emesis basins and seeing the weight loss and the devastation.

Q. *How about the American Cancer Society, should they be the standard for determining what accepted medical use is in the United States?*

A. I think, probably, they have less input.

I think that they are wonderful people, but the American Cancer Society, more than the AMA, is largely lay people, who do wonderful work, but I don't think should be making judgments on how people are treated in the office. I don't think that lies within their domain.

Q. *Going back to the immuno-suppressant side effect that the government mentioned. Have you seen any other side effects from your patient's use of marijuana?*

A. I think probably the only side effect I've seen, that I could even know, would be sedation. Patients will be drowsy.

Q. Would you characterize that as mild or severe. How would you characterize that?

A. Generally it's mild as opposed to oral drugs. A smoked drug is titratable, and patients quickly learn how much they need to relieve the nausea. And that's the key. You can stop [smoking] at the point that the nausea stops and you're through.

Q. How about the euphoric effect that's been attributed to marijuana? Have you - what impact have you seen that have, if any?

A. I am not sure I ever really evaluate that. That would require a complex psychologic study, I suspect.

Somebody who gets treatment, who goes through 12 weeks of drugs in my office who doesn't throw up I suspect, would be euphoric, just because he didn't throw up. I'm not sure it's the direct effect of the drug.

Q. You mentioned the phrase "titration," a second ago, and the government asked you quite a bit about potency of marijuana and so forth. What is titration and how does that impact upon your opinion of marijuana's accepted medical use?

A. Titration is a chemical word. You may have had a chemistry class where you dripped something into acid, into a base and had an indicator that changed color when you got to neutral, or whatever you were doing.

And, you could have the concentration of the acid, and calculate out that you needed twice as much to get the same effect.

Titration, simply, in the patients, means that they realize that if they get a particular preparation that's very potent, they don't need much. If they get a preparation that is not so potent, they need a lot.

As opposed to oral medications which involve no titration. The only titration is whether you absorb it or not, whether you throw it up or not, and that is not titratable. Once you've taken the capsule, it either stays down or doesn't, it gets in your body or it doesn't.

With an inhaled substance and, by the way, this is by no means unique. Having an asthmatic son, he titrates himself with his anti-asthma drugs just by breathing them in. This is a common form of delivering medications, not something rare.

There are many medicines that are delivered by inhalation. And the patients learn to titrate them. They learn how much it takes to stop the nausea and vomiting every bit as much as my son is learning how much anti-asthma medicine he needs to stop his asthmatic attack.

If the manufacturer made four different samples, or four different stock sizes, I suspect my kid is bright enough to learn the difference between them, and when he needs more and when he has had enough. And I think that most patients know that, too.

The patients in my office, in my experience, are not smoking to get high, to get euphoric, to freak out, to jump from roof to roof. They're smoking marijuana to get relief of suffering, which is really what medical oncology is about.

Q. Doctor, during your cross-examination, the subject of in-hospital use versus home use came up. Can you explain to me what you mean, and how does this affect marijuana's use? Where does this factor in to that?

A. Well, the use of anti-nausea medications in complex programs are technically impossible in the setting of private practice.

Marijuana is not technically impossible. The impact—again, going back to a young, gay man with lymphoma who gets 12 treatments—if I had to hospitalize him over night I would basically take somebody with a median survival of less than six months, put them in the hospital, at somebody's cost, we're not concerned about economics, for a minimum of two days. One day in, one day to get his treatment, and the next day to go home. So he's lost all or part of two days.

Twelve treatments, assuming he got nauseated for each treatment and maybe he doesn't, but you don't know that. Twenty four hospital days in somebody who has a survival — a median survival —of less than six months. I've taken one month of his life away, nearly, to give him in-hospital treatment.

These same patients manage themselves at home with marijuana and have that extra 24 days to be with their loved ones.

Q. Doctor, you referred earlier to the acceptance of marijuana in the medical community. Who is in the medical community? What would you define the medical community as?

A. My peers. The people that I share call with, the people that I go to conferences with, not just in San Francisco, but in Los Angeles and San Diego, and in New York and everywhere I go.

Q. How do patients factor into that? Do they constitute part of the medical community as well, or is that a separate community?

A. Well, I think that they're probably separate communities. We listen to what patients say. We try and interact with our patients. And if our patients begin to tell us repetitively that something works, like with the street drugs for AIDS, after we've heard this a couple of times, we may go and say to our colleagues, "Have you heard the same stories?" And when we begin all to hear the same stories, we begin to see whether it has some substance.

But there are clearly, I think, two levels. We talk as physicians, but our patients also talk to us, and I think they're both levels of valid, albeit not published, research.

Q Is that your experience then with marijuana?

A. It is.

Q. Just a couple of more questions for you, Doctor. Do you feel patients accept marijuana as medicine?

A. Not totally. San Francisco, and again I can only speak totally for this community, San Francisco is a heterogeneous community. Because it has been, again my practice is dominantly, although not exclusively gay, because San Francisco has been supportive to the gay life style, many people come from many different areas. And I get people that come from very strict areas of the South and the Midwest. And many of these people have grown up with strong feelings.

The government says that this is the demon weed and you can't use it. And there are patients who are frightened away by that.

There are patients who have detente with their family, even though they have broken out of the mainstream of what we regard as socially acceptable, whose families will sit there and say, "You know, you cannot use such and such a substance." You know, you sit there with the family and you see the mother look horrified when you are talking to her boy about, you know, Compazine doesn't work, Reglan doesn't work. What else do you do and you know what she's thinking or she may actually say about the use of marijuana, because it's illegal. It has that connotation. It's against the law.

Q. Is that why John wouldn't use marijuana?

A. Oh, yeah. John's a Southerner—was a Southerner. He worked for the government in the Forest Service, and was just Mr. Straight Arrow

Q. Just two last questions. Doctor, do you think marijuana has an accepted medical use in the United States?

A. I do.

Q. Do you think marijuana is safe and effective under medical supervision?

A. I do.

Q. No further questions.

III. THE ISSUES

*Can marijuana harm the immune sys-
tem? Is the "pot pill" as effective as natural
marijuana? These are two major issues that
people with AIDS (PWAs) must confront
when considering whether or not to use
marijuana medically. This section explores
those questions.*

Chapter Six
_____

THE IMMUNE QUESTION

The marijuana cigarette has effects that are potentially dangerous including reduced immune deficiency."

> Lee Dogoloff, Executive Director
> American Council for Drug
> Education, on "Sonya Live",
> Cable News Network, July 3, 1991

No significant alterations in immune function tests were observed.

> Elizabeth M. Dax, *et. al.*,
> Reporting on the effects of
> marijuana on the human im-
> mune system. *Journal of Steroid
> Biochemistry*, 1989.

Perhaps one of the most important questions for an HIV+ individual who uses marijuana medically is the question of immune
system effects from the drug.

In the early- and mid-1970s, articles appeared in the press which
alleged marijuana could "damage" the human immune system. The
studies were seriously flawed, as Dr. Leo Hollister explains in the next
chapter, but the press never bothered to look closely at the data and
the ultimate goal—alarming the public about marijuana—was
achieved. Despite an inability by the federal government to replicate
these studies, some federal officials still insist that marijuana can
"damage" the immune system.

More moderate federal officials will talk about marijuana's ability
to "affect" the immune system. While more accurate, even this term
is alarmist, implying a danger that has not been demonstrated.

In America today there are more than 20 million *regular* marijuana smokers. Many of these regular smokers have used the drug since the late-1960s or early-1970s. Yet there is no epidemiological evidence of immune system damage from marijuana use. As Dr. Hollister notes:

> Clinically, one might assume that sustained impairment of cell-mediated immunity [from marijuana smoking] might lead to an increased prevalence of opportunistic infections, or an increased prevalence of malignancy, as seen in the current epidemic of acquired immune deficiency syndrome (AIDS). No such clinical evidence has been discovered nor has any direct epidemiological data incriminated marijuana use with the acquisition of human immunodeficiency virus infection or the clinical development of AIDS.[1]

A federally-funded study by Vera Rubin and Lambros Comitas in the early-1970s looked at the long-term effects of "ganja" or marijuana smoking on the Jamaican population—a culture where marijuana use has long been tolerated and encouraged. It was an ambitious project involving two governments, 60 subjects, and more than 45 professionals. Jamaica was chosen because of widespread marijuana use in the working class. The goal of the study was to gauge the general biological effects of chronic or long-term marijuana smoking.

While not concentrating specifically on immunological effects, Dr. Rubin and Comitas carefully examined the health of their subjects. They reported:

> No serious disease was detected, except for one case of hypertension, and there were no evident signs of nutritional deficiencies. Hemoglobin levels were adequate and serum protein values (albumin and globulin) fell within normal limits. Intestinal parasites, when present, resulted in only light infections. These examinations indicate that ganja smoking does not affect general physical health..."[2]

Despite the work of Rubin and Comitas, U.S. officials continued to insist that marijuana "harmed" the immune system. These claims were based on studies conducted with extremely high doses of syn-

---

1   See Chapter 7, *Marijuana & Immunity.*

2   *Ganja in Jamaica,* Vera Rubin and Lambros Comitas, Mouton & Co. Publishers, The Hague, Paris, pg. 78. 1974

thetic delta-9-tetrahydrocannabinol (THC) — marijuana's psychoactive ingredient—and were conducted using laboratory animals or test tubes. Several small studies involving long-term marijuana smokers were conducted in the mid-1970s. These studies found no difference in the immune system of marijuana smokers. In 1988, the federal government authorized a team of experts from several federal agencies to study the effects of smoked marijuana on the human immune system. Seventeen subjects were entered in the double blind, randomized study. After a two week abstinence from marijuana, the subjects received oral THC or placebo. Several of the subjects also received marijuana cigarettes. The researchers were unable to detect any differences in baseline values of lymphocyte functions, plasma prolactin, adrenocorticotropic hormone (ACTH), cortisol, luteinizing hormones, or testosterone.

The results of the study were published in 1989. Despite the expenditure of federal funds, the use of federal employees in conducting the study, and the authorization of federal authorities to proceed with the study, the results of these experiments have not been aggressively dispensed to other federal agencies. As late as June 1991, federal officials were still claiming marijuana could harm the immune system.

The 1988 study was conducted by professionals of the Addiction Research Center, National Institute on Drug Abuse, and the Clinical Immunology Laboratory, Gerontology Research Center, National Institute on Aging. Previous studies involving humans had used oral THC. The results are definitive.

> "We were unable to demonstrate alterations in tests of lymphocyte function on exposing subjects to psychoactive doses of THC. This is the first report of lymphocyte subset investigations in humans following controlled administration of THC and no alterations were observed. Since no significant alterations were observed either in the acutely treated subjects or in those reporting heavy THC use, we suggest that at least some of the previously described immunosuppressive effects of THC may be nonspecific effects secondary to very high doses of THC used for study."[3]

---

3   "The Effects of 9-ENE-Tetrahydrocannabinol on Hormone Release and Immune Function," *Journal of Steroid Biochemistry*, Vol 34. Nos. 1-6, 1989, pp. 263-270.

In the following chapter Dr. Leo Hollister, professor of Psychiatry and Pharmacology at the University of Texas Medical School in Houston and trustee to the United States Pharmacopeial Convention 1985-1990, offers an overview of previous studies of marijuana's effects on the immune system. Dr. Hollister notes at the onset:

> Few areas of scientific research have been as controversial as the effect of marijuana on immune defenses. The effects of marijuana on health in general have been marked by polarities of belief or interpretation of evidence often due to the particular prejudices of investigators. In addition, evidence of altered immune functions is derived mainly from *in vitro* tests or *ex vivo* experiments, which employed doses of cannabinoids far in excess of those that prevail during social use of marijuana. Finally, the clinical significance of the experimental observations is difficult to assess.

He concludes:

> The relationship between the use of social drugs and the development of clinical manifestations of AIDS has been of some interest, however. Persons infected with the virus but not diagnosed as AIDS have been told to avoid the use of marijuana and/or alcohol. This advice may be reasonable as a general health measure, but direct evidence that heeding this warning will prevent the ultimate damage to the immune system is totally lacking.

For the person with AIDS or HIV infection who is smoking marijuana the real question is not whether marijuana will harm the immune system but rather what is the purity of supply. Illegal marijuana—often purchased from strangers under stressful situations—is subject to all manner of contaminants from natural causes such as fungus and mold. An additional concern is added contaminants such as "angel dust" or other drugs. This makes the case for legal, prescribed marijuana even more compelling. In the meanwhile patients should take care to "know their dealer" and follow the advice of one doctor who advised his patient to "zap" all marijuana supplies in the microwave oven for a brief period of time.

Chapter Seven

MARIJUANA & IMMUNITY*

by Leo Hollister, M.D.

Persons infected with the virus but not diagnosed as AIDS have been told to avoid the use of marijuana and/or alcohol. This advice may be reasonable as a general health measure, but direct evidence that heeding this warning will prevent the ultimate damage to the immune system is totally lacking.

F ew areas of scientific research have been as controversial as the effect of marijuana on immune defenses. The effects of marijuana on health in general have been marked by polarities of belief or interpretation of evidence often due to the particular prejudices of investigators. In addition, evidence of altered immune functions is derived mainly from *in vitro* tests or *ex vivo* experiments, which employed doses of cannabinoids far in excess of those that prevail during social use of marijuana. Finally, the clinical significance of the experimental observations is difficult to assess.

The present review will attempt to objectively assess the evidence. Other recent reviews of the subject have also appeared, with varying degrees of intensity of coverage (Hollister 1986; Maykut 1985; Munson & Fehr 1983; Rosenkrantz 1976). For purposes of a more systematic discussion, immunity will be considered as several separate topics: 1) cell-mediated immunity, 2) humoral mechanisms, 3) cellular defenses, and 4) immunogenicity of marijuana or cannabinoids.

---

* Originally appeared in the *Journal of Psychoactive Drugs*, Volume 20:1, January-March 1988. Reprinted with permission.

CELL-MEDIATED IMMUNITY

Lymphocyte Transformation

Lymphocytes exposed to several mitogens divide rapidly, increase protein and nucleic acid synthesis, and show morphological changes resembling blasts. This test of the ability of T-lymphocytes to transform themselves measures one potential aspect of cell-mediated immunity. A direct way to measure the activation of lymphocytes is to measure the rate of incorporation of a nucleic acid, such as ^{3}H-thymidine, into the cells following addition of the mitogen to the culture. All studies are conducted *in vitro*. An early study (Nahas *et al.* 1976) measured ^{3}H-thymidine uptake in normal human lymphocytes stimulated by both phytohemagglutinin (PHA) and allogenic cell-mixed lymphocyte culture (MLC). The incorporation of ^{3}H-thymidine was equally inhibited by 10^{-5}M to 10^{-4}M concentrations of Δ^9-tetrahydrocannabinol (THC), Δ^8-tetrahydrocannabinol (Δ^8-THC), their corresponding 11-OH metabolites, a variety of other inactive cannabinoids, and olivetol. THC in similar concentrations also depressed ^{3}H-leucine and ^{3}H-uridine uptake, indicating an effect of protein and ribonucleic acid (RNA) synthesis as well. These concentrations of THC were 10 to 20 times greater than those reported earlier by the same group (Nahas *et al.* 1974) as having similar effects. In this study, cell-mediated immunity was evaluated in 51 young, chronic marijuana smokers whose lymphocytes were stimulated *in vitro* by PHA and MLC. As compared with normal controls, ^{3}H-thymidine uptake was reduced.

Klein and colleagues (1985) added the predominantly T-cell mitogens, PHA and concanavalin A (Con A), and the B-cell mitogen, *E. coli* lipopolysaccharide (LPS), to mice spleen cells treated with varying concentrations of THC and its active metabolite 11-OH-THC. Both T-lymphocyte and B-lymphocyte proliferation in response to mitogens were suppressed by THC, but considerably less by 11-OH-THC. Proliferation of both types of lymphocytes was completely inhibited by concentrations of THC (10 μg/ml) that were not directly lytic to the cells. Lower concentrations of THC were found to inhibit B-lymphocytes than those required for T-lymphocytes, suggesting that humoral immunity was more impaired than cell-mediated immunity in this system.

By no means have all studies of cell-mediated immunity in marijuana smokers or *in vitro* exposure of T cells to cannabinoids —often conducted in exactly the same way—shown evidence of immunosuppression. Indeed, the inconsistency of study findings has led to the present state of ambiguity.

White, Brin, and Janicki (1975) obtained peripheral blood lymphocytes from 12 healthy long-term marijuana smokers. The blastogenic response to PHA and pokeweed mitogen were measured *in vitro* by ^{3}H-thymidine uptake. The responses of lymphocytes from the marijuana smokers were not significantly different from those who did not smoke the drug.

Lau and colleagues (1976) observed 8 chronic smokers of marijuana in a hospital setting over a 30-day period. Each subject received a placebo during the first 6 days, followed by THC in oral doses up to 210 mg/day for the next 18 days, and then a placebo for the last 6 days. The response of their lymphocytes to PHA stimulation, as measured by ^{3}H-thymidine uptake, was no different in either of the three periods.

Rachelfsky and Opedz (1977) stimulated normal human lymphocytes with PHA and with MLC, and ^{3}H-thymidine uptake was measured. The uptake of thymidine was unchanged in lymphocytes exposed to 1.9×10^{-4}M or 12.0×10^{-4}M concentrations of THC. Higher concentrations of THC precipitated in the medium. Changes were comparable in cells exposed to THC and in those not so exposed. Kakiamani and colleagues (1978) obtained peripheral lymphocytes from 12 chronic users of marijuana and 15 nonusing control subjects. Lymphocytes from the experienced marijuana users were obtained both before and after smoking hashish. Incorporation of ^{14}C-thymidine, after PHA stimulation and formation of rosettes of sheep erythrocytes, was no different between the normal controls and the marijuana users either before or after the latter had smoked hashish.

Whatever immunosuppressive effects marijuana may have, they are not dependent on psychoactive components. A variety of cannabinoids which have no apparent central nervous system activity, share an apparent immunosuppressive action (Smith *et al.* 1978).

T-Lymphocyte Rosette Formation

Another commonly used measure of cell-mediated immunity is the ability of T-lymphocytes to form *in vitro* rosettes of sheep erythrocytes surrounding T cells. A dose-related decrease in rosette formation was found in sensitized T cells exposed *in vitro* to various concentrations or THC in this medium (Cushman, Khurana, & Hashim 1976).Cushman and Khwana (1977) tested 10 subjects during a 4 week cycle of marijuana smoking, so that the subjects were exposed chronically rather than acutely, and the results showed a decrease in early T-cell rosette formation but no change in either late T-cell or B-cell rosettes. When Gupta, Grieco, and Cushman (1974) compared 23 chronic marijuana smokers with 23 nonsmokers, T-cell rosettes were decreased in the users as compared with the nonusers but rosettes associated with B-lymphocytes were not different, suggesting a selective effect on cell-mediated immunity.

Petersen, Grahan, and Lemberger (1976) tested three subjects who smoked "street" marijuana for rosette formation and blastogenesis. Two of the three showed decreased rosette formation and impaired blastogenesis following stimulation of their lymphocytes with PHA. In another trial, rosette formation was measured in 6 persons 3 to 6 hours after they smoked a marijuana cigarette containing 10 mg of THC. Rosette formation was impaired in 5 of the subjects, and became normal 24 hours later in all but one subject. Thus, it appeared that the effects of marijuana on T-lymphocytes are variable and reversible, suggesting that factors other than exposure to marijuana itself may be involved.

Mice immunized with sheep erythrocytes were treated with intraperitoneal doses of 10, 25, and 40 mg/kg/day of THC for 7 to 8 days. Both plaque-forming and rosette-forming cells were decreased by the 25 mg/kg/day dose (Lefkowitz et al. 1978). Monkeys were exposed to three levels of marijuana smoke over a six-month period. Plasma immunoglobulin (IgG and IgM) were decreased in those monkeys exposed to medium and high concentrations of smoke. In vitro tests by Dual and Heath (1975) of the response of lymphocytes to Con A were decreased. Thus, both humoral and cell-mediated immunity appeared to be affected. However, the authors asserted that it is impossible to assess the in vivo implications from tests of this sort.

Cushman and Khurana (1977) tested 10 subjects during a 4 week cycle of marijuana smoking, so that the subjects were exposed chronically rather than acutely. The results showed a decrease in early T-cell rosette formation, but no change in either late T-cell or B-cell rosettes.

These studies also indicated that T-lymphocyte function, as measured by rosette formation, was decreased when the cells are exposed to cannabinoids either in vitro or ex vivo. However, these impairments were rapidly reversible.

Other Measurements of Cell-Mediated Immunity

A number of other measurements of cell-mediated immunity have pointed in the same direction. Although both impaired allograft rejection and decreased hemagglutinin titers were found in animals treated with cannabinoids, the effect on allograft rejection as a measure of cell-mediated immunity was greater (Munson et al. 1976). Susceptibility to infection with herpes simplex virus type 2 applied directly to the vagina was increased in mice that had received doses of 100 mg/kg/day of THC (Mishkin & Cabral 1985). A similar increased susceptibility was found in guinea pigs treated with doses of 4.0 and 10 mg/kg/day (Cabral *et al.* 1986).

Morohan and colleagues assessed the LD_{50} dose of *Listeria monocytogenes* in mice treated with THC in doses of 38, 75, and 150 mg/kg. The LD_{50} was decreased 10- 17-and 657-fold by each dose, respectively. Marijuana extract was less active. A similar challenge with herpes simplex type 2 virus showed a 96-fold decrease following administration of THC, with no decreased resistance following administration of marijuana extract. These situations are not at all comparable to human exposure.

The vast majority of people can be made sensitive to dinitrochlorobenzene (DNCB), a powerful skin sensitizer. DNCB is often used with "recall" antigens (*e.g.*, tuberculin and mumps) to test patients for anergy. Sensitivity to DNCB was found in all 34 chronic marijuana smokers who were tested as compared with 96% of 279 healthy nonsmokers. On the other hand, 34 patients with cancer, whose cell-mediated immunity is sometimes decreased, showed a positive reaction in only 70% of those tested (Silverstein & Lessin 1974). Such evidence raises questions about the clinical significance of experiments that have shown evidence of cell-mediated immunity from cannabinoids.

It has been hypothesized that the membrane-disordering effects of THC may affect the binding of antigens to cellular receptors, accounting for a decrease in cell-mediated immunity. On the other hand, the combination of increased membrane disorder and inhibition of acyltransferase activity in B cells and T cells could impair the transfer of cellular constituents (Baczynsky & Zimmerman 1983b). Regardless of whether the action is a nonspecific one at the cell membrane or at a more primary site, impaired immunity remains precisely that. However, a cell membrane site of action could explain the apparent transitory nature of the observed alterations in cell-mediated immunity as well as the requirement for much larger concentrations of cannabinoids than those usually encountered during social use of marijuana.

Summary of Effects of Cell-Mediated Immunity

In summary, the effects of cannabinoids on cell-mediated immunity are contradictory. Such evidence as has been obtained to support such an effect has usually involved doses and concentrations that are orders of magnitude greater than those obtained when marijuana is used by human subjects. Clinically, one might assume that sustained impairment of cell-mediated immunity might lead to an increased prevalence of opportunistic infections, or an increased prevalence of malignancy, as seen in the current epidemic of acquired immune deficiency syndrome (AIDS). No such clinical evidence has been discovered or has any direct epidemiological data incriminated marijuana use with the acquisition of human immunodeficiency virus infection or the clinical development of AIDS. Even though some degree of impairment of immune responses were to occur, the remaining immune function may be adequate, especially in the young persons who are the major users of cannabis.

HUMORAL IMMUNITY

Transformation of B-lymphocytes

Transformation of B cells stimulated by the mitogen LPS was inhibited more than were T cells stimulated by PHA following the same doses of THC in mice (Klein *et al.* 1985). This evidence of diminished B-cell reactivity following the administration of THC was confirmed in another study (Munson *et al.* 1976) that showed a dose-dependent suppression from doses of 50, 100, and 200 mg/kg of THC in mice. These doses are enormous, of course.

Antibody Formation

A frequently used measure of humoral immunity is the ability of splenic lymphocytes from mice that are immunized against sheep erythrocytes to form plaques when exposed *in vitro* to sheep erythrocytes. Levy and Heppner (1981) found that both THC and haloperidol produced dose-dependent reductions in hemolytic plaque-forming cell (PFC) numbers at the time of peak reactivity (day 4) in control mice. Treatment with THC and haloperidol only delayed the time of peak PFC formation by 24 to 48 hours (doses were high enough to produce signs of gross behavioral toxicity). Neither THC nor other cannabinoids had any effect on the titer of serum hemagglutinating antibody measured 7 days after immunization.

Baczynsky and Zimmerman (1983a) immunized mice with sheep erythrocytes on Day 1 (primary immune response) and on days 1 and 28 (secondary immune response) and measured hemagglutinin titers. Mice treated with 10 or 15 mg of THC during the primary immunization period exhibited a suppression of the primary humoral immune response. These doses also suppressed the secondary immune response, even when given during the period of primary immunization. Mice treated with THC during the secondary immunization period showed no measurable response. Other cannabinoids had no effect.

Immature mice immunized with sheep erythrocytes also showed suppression of the immune response when treated with THC in doses of 1.0, 5.0, and 10.0 mg/kg. Splenic weight was reduced and PFC as well as hemagglutinin titers were lower than controls. The suppression was specific for THC and was not observed with cannabidiol or cannabinol, even at doses of 25 mg/kg (Zimmerman et al. 1977). Some evidence of tolerance or hyporesponsiveness to this humoral antibody suppression by THC was found when mice were treated with THC for five days prior to immunization as well as afterward (Loveless, Harris, & Munson 1981-1982).

Rosenkrantz, Miller, and Esber (1975) immunized rats with a single intraperitoneal dose of sheep erythrocytes during, before, and after administration of THC in order to determine its effect on the inductive and productive phases of the primary immune response. Following a dose of 10 mg/kg, THC decreased the primary immune response by 33 to 40%; the inductive phase was decreased by 48 to 78% by all doses of THC, and the productive phase was decreased by 26 to 59% by the higher doses.

The same group (Luthra et al. 1980) tested the primary immune response of rats to intraperitoneal administration of sheep erythrocytes after 5 to 26 days following pretreatment with THC in order to determine if tolerance developed to the immunosuppressant effects. As measured by splenic antibody-forming cells and hemagglutinin/hemolysin titers, no evidence of tolerance was found.

Summary of Effects of Humoral Immunity

In summary, humoral immunity, as tested by a number of *in vitro* procedures, seems also to be impaired by cannabinoids, but this effect was most evident for THC. The clinical significance of such changes is questionable due to the great concentrations of cannabinoids used and the lack of any epidemiological evidence of increased bacterial infections in chronic users of marijuana.

CELLULAR DEFENSES

Leukocytes and Lymphocytes

When 10 subjects were followed through a 4 week cycle of marijuana smoking, no change was observed either in peripheral leukocyte or absolute lymphocyte counts (Cushman & Khwana 1977). Leukocytes from 5 chronic marijuana smokers were compared with those from 5 nonusers of the drug for their ability to migrate after exposure to THC or marijuana extract. Both treatments inhibited leukocyte migration without killing the cells, both in cells from users and nonusers of marijuana. The prevailing THC concentration needed to accomplish this was 2.0 mg/ml, a couple of orders of magnitude greater than any THC plasma concentrations usually found clinically (Schwartzfarb, Needle, & Chavez-Chase 1974).

Natural Killer-Cell Activity

Natural killer-cell activity in rats was decreased by subchronic treatment (25 days) with THC, but not after acute treatment (1 day). This effect was not found in rats treated simultaneously with naloxone, suggesting possible involvement of the opiate system (Patel *et al.* 1985). When injected into mice, both THC and its active metabolite 11-OH-THC suppressed splenic natural killer-cell activity *in vitro*. The tissue concentrations of the cannabinoids were reported as being 5.0-10.0 mg/ml, about two orders of magnitude greater than those that might be experienced during the social use of marijuana (Klein, Newton, & Friedman 1987).

Macrophages

Macrophages work closely with T cells as part of the immunological defense system. On glass surfaces, macrophage cultures normally show spreading, which is an indication of their mobility. The addition of THC to the medium inhibited the degree of spreading. It also inhibited the phagocytosis of yeast particles (Lopez-Cepero *et al.* 1986). However, another experiment (Munsan *et al.* 1976) using intact mice that were treated with a single dose or multiple doses of THC could not demonstrate impairment in reticuloendothelial activity, as measured by the intravascular clearance of colloidal carbon.

Summary of Effects on Cellular Defenses

It is somewhat surprising that newer techniques of cell sorting, which permit determination of absolute counts of T- and B-lymphocytes as well as subsets of T-lymphocytes, have not been utilized. The evidence from the *in vitro* studies is weakened by the high concentrations of drug that were used. Clinically, evidence for impairment of cellular defenses has not been forthcoming.

IMMUNOGENICITY OF CANNABINOIDS

Laboratory Studies

It has been hypothesized that THC, a relatively simple chemical, can act as a hapten and become an immunogen. If such were the case, tolerance to THC might be explained on an immunological basis as well as the rare reports of allergic reactions. Azathioprine, an immunosuppressant, had a modest effect in mitigating the hypotensive effects of THC in spontaneously hypertensive rats. Spleen cells from mice treated with THC showed slightly more blast transformation in culture than untreated spleen cells, either with or without THC being added to the culture medium. However, the degree of blast transformation was far less than that produced by PHA. This somewhat weak evidence for an immunogenic action of THC came from a laboratory that later stressed the immunosuppressant effects of marijuana (Nahas, Zugury, & Sehwartz 1973).

Watson, Murphy, & Tumer (1983) employed a technique used to test compounds for their potential for producing allergic contact dermatitis and that also maximizes the degree of skin sensitization of guinea pigs. Sensitivity was greatly increased by THC and cannabinol, but less so with other cannabinoids.

Clinical Studies

In a clinical study conducted in the southwestern United States (Freeman 1983), skin tests were applied to 90 patients with various forms of atopy. The test was positive for 63 patients for marijuana pollen as compared to only 18 who had reacted to tobacco leaf. However, it is unlikely that marijuana pollen contains many cannabinoids, but rather contains proteins that may be sensitizing.

A series of 28 marijuana smokers showed precipitins for *Aspergillus* antigens: 13 were positive as compared to 1 of 10 controls. Lymphocytes showed significant blastogenesis in 3 of those subjects who tested positive. Seven of these 23 subjects reported bronchospasm following the smoking of marijuana, and one patient had evidence of systemic aspergillosis (Kagen *et al.* 1983). As it is well known that marijuana contains contaminants, including molds and fungi, it is not surprising that these should cause allergic reactions in some users. The study does not indicate that cannabinoids themselves are immunogens.

Skin testing with cannabinoids seems to be useless for determining the rare patient with sensitivity to marijuana. A variety of intradermal tests with various cannabinoids and common allergens was applied to 63 marijuana users by Lewis and Slavin (1971). Two users, who were clearly atopic with a past history of bronchial asthma, also reported experiencing asthma after some exposures to marijuana. A third subject, with a history of allergic rhinitis, also experienced similar symptoms following marijuana use. All three of these subjects had negative skin tests to cannabinoids. On the other hand, 7 subjects who tested positive for hemp and one who tested positive to Δ^8-THC had no clinical manifestation of marijuana sensitivity.

A 29-year-old woman (known to be allergic to ragweed) experienced symptoms of an anaphylactoid reaction that lasted 20 to 30 minutes immediately after smoking marijuana. Skin tests with THC showed a 2+ reaction, and with cannabidiol a 1+ reaction (Liskow, Liss, & Parker 1971). The weakly positive skin tests do not necessarily indicate that the reaction was due specifically to the cannabinoids.

Summary of Immunogenicity

While it is possible that a few persons may become truly allergic to cannabinoids, it is far more likely that allergic reactions, which have been exceedingly rare following the use of marijuana, are due to contaminants. Marijuana is grown in the field and harvested along with everything else (*e.g.*, bacteria, fungi, molds, parasites, worms, chemicals) that may be found in such field plants. That such impure material, when smoked and inhaled into the lungs, causes so little trouble is really a marvel.

SUMMARY AND CONCLUSIONS

Despite the fairly large volume of literature that developed during the past 15 years or so, the effect of cannabinoids on the immune system is still unsettled. The evidence has been contradictory and is more supportive of some degree of immunosuppression only when one considers *in vitro* studies. These have been seriously flawed by the very high concentrations of drug used to produce immunosuppression and by the lack of comparisons with other membrane active drugs. The closer that experimental studies have been to actual clinical situations, the less compelling has been the evidence.

Although the topic was of great interest during the 1970s, as indicated by the preponderance of the references from that period, interest has waned during the present decade. This waning of interest suggests that perhaps most investigators feel that this line of inquiry will not be rewarding. The AIDS epidemic has also diverted the attention of immunologists to the far more serious problem of the truly devastating effects a retrovirus can have on a portion of the immune system.

The relationship between the use of social drugs and the development of clinical manifestations of AIDS has been of some interest, however. Persons infected with the virus but not diagnosed as AIDS have been told to avoid the use of marijuana and/or alcohol. This advice may be reasonable as a general health measure, but direct evidence that heeding this warning will prevent the ultimate damage to the immune system is totally lacking.

ACKNOWLEDGMENTS

The author wishes to thank Matthew Edlund, M.D., who provided useful critical comments during the preparation of this article.

REFERENCES

Baczynsky, W.O. & Zimmerman, A.M. "Effects of Δ^9-tetrahydrocannabinol, cannabinol and cannabidiol on the immune system of mice. I. *In vivo* investigation of the primary and secondary immune response." *Pharmacology*, Vol. 26(1):1-11, 1983a.

Baczynsky, W.O. & Zimmerman, A.M. "Effects of Δ^9-tetrahydrocannabinol, cannabinol and cannabidiol on the immune system of mice. II. *In vitro* investigation using cultured mouse splenocytes." *Pharmacology*, Vol. 26(1): 12-19, 1983b.

Bradley, S.G.; Munson, A.E.; Dewey, W.L. & Harris, L.S. "Enhanced susceptibility of mice to combinations of Δ^9-tetrahydrocannabinol and live or killed gram negative bacteria." *Infection and Immunity*, Vol. 17: 325-329, 1977.

Cabral, G.A.; Mishkin, E.M.; Marciano-Cabral, F.; Coleman, P.; Harris, L. & Munson, A.E. "Effect of Δ^9-tetrahydrocannabinol on herpes simplex virus type 2 vaginal infection in the guinea pig." *Proceedings of the Society for Experimental Biology and Medicine*, Vol. 182: 181-186, 1986.

Cushman, P. & Khurana, R. "A controlled cycle of tetrahydrocannabinol smoking: T and B cell rosette formation." *Life Sciences*, Vol. 20: 971-980, 1977.

Cushman, P.; Khurana, R. & Hashim, G. "Tetrahydrocannabinol: Evidence for reduced rosette formation by normal T lymphocytes." In: Braude, M.C. & Szara, S. (Eds.). *The Pharmacology of Marihuana*. Raven Press:New York, 1976.

Dual, C.B. & Heath, R.G. "The effect of chronic marihuana usage on the immunological status of rhesus monkeys." *Life Sciences*, Vol. 17: 875, 1975.

Freeman, G.L. "Allergic skin test reactivity to marijuana in the Southwest." *Western Journal of Medicine*, Vol. 138(6): 829-831, 1983.

Gupta, S.; Grieco, M.A. & Cushman, P. "Impairment of rosette forming T lymphocytes in chronic marihuana smokers." *New England Journal of Medicine*, Vol. 291: 874-877, 1974.

Hollister, L.E. "Health aspects of cannabis." *Pharmacological Reviews*, Vol. 38(1): 1-20, 1986.

Kagen, S.L.; Kurup, V.P.; Sohnle, P.G. & Fink, J.N. "Marijuana smoking and fungal sensitization." *Journal of Allergy and Clinical Immunology*, Vol. 71 (4): 389-393, 1983.

Kaklamani, E.; Trichopoulos, D.;Koutselinis, A.;Brouja, M. & Karalis, B. "Hashish smoking and T-lymphocytes." *Archives of Toxicology*, Vol. 40: 97-101, 1978.

Klein, T.W.; Newton, C. & Friedman, H. "Inhibition of natural killer cell function by marijuana components." *Journal of Toxicology and Environmental Health*, Vol. 20(4): 321-332, 1987.

Klein, T.W.; Newton, C.; Widen, R. & Friedman, H. "The effect of Δ^9-tetrahydrocannabinol and 11-hydroxy-Δ^9-tetrahydrocannabinol on T-lymphocyte and B-lymphocyte mitogen responses." *Journal of Immunopharmacology*, Vol. 7: 451-456, 1985.

Lau, R.J.; Tubergen, D.G.; Barr, M., JR.; Domino, E.F.; Benowitz, N. & Jones, R.T. "Phytohemagglutinin-induced lymphocyte transformation in humans receiving Δ^9-tetrahydrocannabinol." *Science*, Vol. 192: 805-807, 1976.

Lefkowitz, S.S.; Klager, K.; Nemeth, D. & Pruess, M. "Immunosuppression of mice by Δ^9-THC." *Research Communications in Chemical Pathology and Pharmacology*, Vol. 19: 101-107, 1978.

Levy, J.A. & Heppner, G.H. "Alterations of immune reactivity by haloperidol and Δ^9-tetrahydrocannabinol." *Journal of Immunopharmacology*, Vol 3:93-109, 1981.

Levy, J.A.; Munson, A.E.; Harris, L.S. & Dewey, W.L. "Effect of Δ^8-and Δ^9-tetrahydrocannabinol on the immune response in mice." *Pharmacologist*, Vol. 16: 259, 1974.

Lewis, C.R. & Slavin, R.G. "Allergy to marihuana: A clinical and skin-testing study." *Journal of Allergy and Clinical Immunology*, Vol. 55: 131-132, 1975.

Liskow, D.; Liss, J.L. & Parker, C.W. "Allergy to marihuana." *Annals of Internal Medicine*, Vol. 75: 571-573, 1971.

Lopez-Cepero, M.; Friedman, M.; Klein, T. & Friedman, H. "Tetrahydrocannabinol-induced suppression of macrophage spreading and phagocyte activity *in vitro*." *Journal of Leukocyte Biology*, Vol. 39: 679-686, 1986.

Loveless, S.E.; Harris, I..S. & Munson, A.E. "Hyporesponsiveness to the immunosuppressant effects of Δ^8-tetrahydrocannabinol." *Journal of Immunopharmacology*, Vol. 3(3-4): 371-383, 1981-1982.

Luthra, Y.K.; Esber, H.J.; Lariviere, D.M. & Rosenkrantz, H. "Assessment of tolerance to immunosuppressive activity of Δ^9-tetrahydrocannabinol in rats." *Journal of Immunopharmacology*, Vol. 2:245, 1980.

Maykut, M.O. "Health consequences of acute and chronic marihuana use." *Progress in Neuropsychopharmarcology and Biological Psychiatry*, Vol. 9(3): 209-238, 1985.

Mishkin, E.M. & Cabral, G.A. "Δ^9-tetrahydrocannabinol decreases host resistance to herpes simplex virus type 2 vaginal infection in the B6C3F1 mouse." *Journal of General Virology*, Vol. 66: 2539-2549, 1985.

Morahan, P.S.; Klykken, P.C.; Smith S.H.; Harris, L.S. & Munson A.E. "Effects of cannabinoids on host resistance to *Listeria monocytogenes* and herpes simplex virus." *Infection and Immunity*, Vol 23:670-674, 1979.

Munson, A.E. & Fehr, K.O. "Immunological effects of cannabis." In: Fehr, K.O. & Kalant, H. (Eds.). *Cannabis and Health Hazards*. Addiction Research Foundation:Toronto, 1983.

Munson, A.E.; Levy, J.A.; Harris, L.S. & Dewey, W.L. "Effects of Δ^9-tetrahydrocannabinol on the immune system." In: Braude M.C. & Szara, S. (Eds.). *The Pharmacology of Marihuana*. Raven Press: New York, 1976.

Nahas, G.G.; Desoize, B.; Armand, I.P.; Hsu. J. & Morishima, A. "Natural cannabinoids: Apparent depression of nucleic acids and protein synthesis in cultured human lymphocytes." In: Braude M.C. & Szara, S. (Eds.). *The Pharmacology of Marihuana*. Raven Press:New York, 1976.

Nahas, G.G.; Suciv-Foca, N.; Armand, J.P. & Morishima, A. "Inhibition of cellular mediated immunity in marihuana smokers." *Science*, Vol. 183: 419-420, 1974.

Nahas, G.G.; Zagury, D. & Schwartz, I.W. "Evidence for the possible immunogenicity of Δ^9-tetrahydrocannabinol (THC) in rodents." *Nature*, Vol. 243: 407-408, 1973.

Patel, V.; Borysendo, M.; Kumar, M.S.A. & Millard, W.J. "Effects of acute and subchronic Δ^9-tetrahydrocannabinol administration on the plasma catecholamine, β–endorphin, and corticosterone levels and splenic natural killer activity in rats." *Proceedings of the Society of Experimental Biology and Medicine*, Vol. 180: 400-404, 1985.

Petersen, B.H.; Grahen, J. & Lemberger, L. "Marihuana, tetrahydrocannabinol, and T-cell function." *Life Sciences*, Vol. 1976: 395-400, 1976.

Rachelfsky, G.S. & Opedz, G. "Normal lymphocyte function in the presence of Δ^9-THC." *Clinical Pharmacology and Therapeutics*, Vol. 21: 44-46, 1977.

Rosenkrantz, H. "The immune response and marihuana." In: Nahas, G. (Ed.). *Marihuana: Chemistry, Biochemistry, and Cellular Effects*. Springer-Verlag:New York, 1976.

Rosenkrantz, H.; Miller, A.J. & Esber, H.J. "Δ^9-tetrahydrocannabinol suppression of the primary immune response in rats." *Journal of Toxicology and Environmental Health*, Vol. 1: 119, 1975.

Schwartzfarb L.; Needle, N. & Chevez-Chase, M. "Dose-related inhibition of leukocyte migration by marijuana and Δ^9-tetrahydrocannabinol." *Journal of Clinical Pharmacology*, Vol. 14: 35-41, 1974.

Silverstein, M.I. & Lessin, P.J. "Normal skin test responses in chronic marijuana users." *Science*, Vol. 186:740-741, 1974.

Smith S.; Harris L.; Uwaydah, I. & Munson, A. "Structure-activity relationships of natural and synthetic cannabinoids in suppression of humoral and cell-mediated immunity." *Journal of Pharmacology and Experimental Therapeutics*, Vol. 207: 165-170, 1978.

Watson, E.S.; Murphy, J.D. & Turner, C.E. "Allergenic properties of naturally occurring cannabinoids." *Journal of Pharmaceutical Sciences*, Vol. 72: 954-955, 1983.

White, S.C.; Brin, S.C. & Janicki, B.W. "Mitogen-induced blastogenic responses of lymphocytes from marihuana smokers." *Science*, Vol. 188: 71-72, 1975.

Zimmerman, S.; Zimmerman, A.M.; Cameron, I.L. & Laurence, H.L. "Δ^9-tetrahydrocannabinol, cannabidiol, and cannabinol effects on the immune response of mice." *Pharmacology*, Vol. 15: 10-23, 1977.

Chapter Eight

MARINOL v. MARIJUANA

"Public Health Service believes that whenever possible [AIDS patients] should use THC (Marinol)—which is reliable, effective, and much less harmful—instead of marijuana.

> Bill Grigg, FDA Spokesperson
> June 21, 1991

My wife tried Marinol and it didn't work. It made her sicker than without the drug....She just couldn't tolerate it. It was an unsafe drug for her.

> Kenny Jenks appearing on
> "Sonya Live," Cable News
> Network, July 3, 1991

On June 21, 1991, the Public Health Service (PHS) announced AIDS patients would no longer be granted compassionate access to marijuana such as that given to Steve, Barbra, Kenny, and Danny. From now on, the PHS declared, AIDS patients would have to use Marinol, a synthetic form of marijuana's psychoactive ingredient delta-9-tetrahydrocannabinol (THC).

The announcement was a devastating blow to hundreds of AIDS patients who had hoped for legal access to marijuana through the Food and Drug Administration (FDA). Many had already tried Marinol and it had not worked. For them the FDA was once again denying them a needed medication. One AIDS patient, when informed of the new policy, replied, "What agency door must I chain myself to now? How can they continue to do this to us?"

Marinol

Marinol was approved for marketing in 1986. It is a synthetic version of marijuana's psychoactive ingredient THC. Marinol is often referred to as the "pot pill" but it is, in fact, only one part of the marijuana plant. It is manufactured by Unimed, Inc, a New Jersey-based pharmaceutical company.

Marinol's release in 1986 was widely heralded by federal officials who hoped the move would derail growing public demands for prescriptive access to marijuana. The pressure was great indeed. Between 1978 and 1983, 34 state legislatures passed bills that recognized the therapeutic value of marijuana in the treatment of glaucoma and the side-effects of cancer chemotherapy. Federal legislation had been proposed in Congress and was gaining a substantial number of co-sponsors. Several courts had upheld the defense of medical necessity and acquitted individuals charged with marijuana possession.

The release of Marinol achieved the desired political effect of slowing calls for reform. Headlines declaring "Marijuana Pill Approved for Medical Use" gave the public an impression that the problem had been resolved. Marijuana was now available by prescription—or so it seemed.

In fact, marijuana was not available at all. Marinol was available, but only in highly restrictive settings. For the glaucoma patient, or those afflicted with multiple sclerosis (MS), chronic pain, paralysis, and other ailments, legal access to marijuana was still out of reach.

Tightly Restricted Use

According to the package insert, "Marinol is indicated for treatment of nausea and vomiting associated with cancer chemotherapy in patients who have failed to respond adequately to conventional antiemetic treatments."

The package insert for Marinol goes on to note, "This restriction is required because a substantial proportion of patients treated with Marinol can be expected to experience disturbing psychotomimetic reactions not observed with other antiemetic agents."

Problems with Marinol (THC) had been noted early in its development. Despite claims from the PHS that THC is "reliable and effective," an internal memorandum from the National Cancer Institute (NCI) in May 1978, notes that the "oral absorption of THC is erratic" and some researchers questioned the wisdom of using an oral medication with vomiting patients. The memorandum concluded that "all in all the [marijuana] cigarette may be the best means of administering the drug."

Nevertheless, it was more politically expedient to release Marinol than to acknowledge the medicinal value of marijuana in its natural state and so Marinol was approved.

Marinol's sales in the late-1980s were respectable but not earth-shattering. Tight restrictions on use of the drug, coupled with the rather chilling comments of the package insert, did little to encourage physicians to use Marinol. Indeed, many oncologists continued to encourage patients to use marijuana, albeit illegally. A Harvard University survey conducted in the spring of 1990 revealed that 55% of America's oncologists found marijuana safe and effective. A whopping 69% had discussed marijuana's medical use with their patients and 44% had recommended the illegal drug to their patients.

Physicians also told Harvard researchers that marijuana was more effective than Marinol.

Marinol's Use with HIV Infection

In approximately 1988, internists who were treating people with HIV infection began to quietly prescribe Marinol to their patients. In many cases, the prescription fell within the tight restrictions approved for Marinol. HIV patients being treated for lymphomas were probably among the first to receive Marinol, but slowly use of the drug was expanded to include patients receiving AZT. The rational was that AZT (or perhaps the disease itself) caused nausea and vomiting which did not respond to conventional antiemetics therefore Marinol could be prescribed.

In fact, many people with AIDS (PWAs) were already smoking marijuana to quell the AZT-induced nausea and vomiting. More importantly, marijuana was stimulating their appetite and helping them maintain body weight. This information was shared with their doctors who quietly made note of the illegal drug's use and began to look upon Marinol as a legal, albeit inferior, alternative.

This information was, in turn, shared with Unimed and its partner Roxanne Laboratories. Anxious to expand its market, Unimed began to pursue studies of the synthetic drug's use in PWAs. A preliminary study with 10 patients was completed in San Francisco in 1990. Unimed reported that 7 patients gained weight and 2 reduced their rate of weight loss. According to the Unimed annual report, "Prior to treatment with Marinol, patients were losing an average of 2 pounds per month. During treatment, this was reversed to an average gain of 1.2 pounds per month." Unimed went on to report that a "separate study revealed that the optimal dose of Marinol increased the appetite of cancer patients." The report concluded that "Appetite stimulation would be an important new indication for Marinol and could expand its market ten-fold."

To further protect its market, Unimed requested and was granted orphan drug status for Marinol as an appetite stimulant and for prevention of weight loss in AIDS patients. Orphan drug status for Marinol guaranteed Unimed seven years of non-competitive marketing for its pill which had been developed at taxpayer expense and was now selling for $8 a tablet.

Marinol v. Marijuana - User Comments

But does Marinol work? While some patients have had success with the synthetic drug an overwhelming number of AIDS patients report Marinol is marginally effective and extremely unreliable.

Jim Barnes of Michigan writes:

> After leaving the hospital at the end of 1989 I began smoking marijuana. The benefit of doing this included relief from nausea and vomiting, increased appetite, and relief of headaches. My doctor was aware of this and understood why I was doing this. As time went on I found it harder and harder to find marijuana and when I did I couldn't afford it. Finally I approached my doctor to see if we could petition the government for medical use of marijuana. He said he was willing but there wasn't any way to do so and even if there was a way the government would say no. He said he could prescribe Marinol.
>
> I am generally very uneasy about taking drugs of any kind and usually do not. As I could not find marijuana I agreed to try Marinol. Overall I was very disappointed with Marinol. Never did it seem to relieve my nausea. Mostly it was a matter of wondering what it was doing to my body as I waited for it to work. It didn't help my appetite much less ease my headaches. Compared with marijuana Marinol is a joke. Immediately after smoking marijuana my nausea would lessen and I'd have an improved appetite. A while later my

headaches would lessen and sometimes stop all
together. From my experience the choice between
Marinol and marijuana is clear—flush the
Marinol down the toilet and have a smoke.[*]

Dan C. of Pennsylvania has a different view of Marinol's effectiveness
but his comments on the drug's side-effects are worrisome.

I've been taking Marinol for almost a year now
and I do find it very helpful. However it isn't always consistent. Sometimes it gives me great appetite, other times it's like I took nothing at all.
Since before my diagnosis I have had nausea and
vomiting. If I do nothing, I have no appetite. I've
gone from 185-190 lbs. to 169 lbs. within a matter of months.

When I started taking Marinol I felt very light-
headed. After a point I am no longer aware of that
feeling. That is to say, the feeling is barely noticeable or nothing at all. What seems more consistent is dryness of mouth. I also believe that it is
extremely habit forming and sometimes if I miss
an occasional dose for too long I get a headache.
However, that's not consistent either.

I have also found that marijuana is much more
consistent than Marinol. Marijuana immediately
creates an appetite. Mostly its effect on nausea is
remarkable. Without creating an appetite it's almost worth its weight in gold getting rid of the
nausea. Sometimes when I'm not nauseous I can
make myself eat without a true appetite. But
without something to aid in this I'm usually nauseous most of the time. Marijuana has been the
most effective thing for me but I rarely have access to any.

Barbra Jenks was given Marinol while hospitalized for a bout of
pneumonia in the Spring of 1991. Her comments:

---

[*]   Editor's note: Jim Barnes' doctor did finally petition the government on
       Jim's behalf with the help of the Alliance for Cannabis Therapeutics. Jim
       received FDA permission to legally smoke marijuana in February 1991.

They brought me my first Marinol pill late in the evening, around 8:30 or 9:00. About midnight my heart suddenly started racing. I could hear and feel it pounding like crazy in my chest. Everything felt speedy. I felt like I was going 100 mph down the highway with no brakes. That's when my whole body started to shake. I began to feel trapped, confined, very claustrophobic.

I tried to remain calm. But the more I tried to sleep the more out of control I felt. I was getting panicky. Really frightened.

These feelings, emotions, thoughts continued for several hours. Then I started having hot flashes. I wanted it to stop. I wanted to be normal. I wanted to be nauseated. I felt like I was going crazy or dying or both.

Breakfast arrived. I was too nauseated to eat. The doctor came in for his morning visit. I told him about my Marinol experience. He seemed to understand. After he left I still couldn't get to sleep. I no longer felt like I was going crazy, but everything seemed on edge.

Lunch came. Still couldn't eat because of nausea. At 2:00 p.m. they brought me my third Marinol pill. I was beginning not to like Marinol.

That afternoon I developed a terrible headache. My shoulders and neck ached and felt stiff, all my joints hurt, my hands felt cramped and arthritic. My whole body was just one dull, endless ache that wouldn't go away.

When they came in to give me my fourth dose I flatout refused to take any more Marinol. I was still nauseated, but most of all I desperately wanted to sleep. So I just said "No more."

I didn't tell the nurses, but I wanted to find out if I was going crazy or if it was Marinol that was causing all these weird, frightening emotions and sensations. Maybe AIDS was affecting my mind. Or my breathing problem was causing me to think crazy. I felt a real anxiety about knowing the answer.

There was a really big difference between how I feel after smoking marijuana and how I feel after taking Marinol. Marijuana makes me feel relaxed. I can think clearly. I don't get very confused. Most important, I don't feel like things are out of control or that I'm going crazy. To be honest, I like how marijuana makes me feel. When I smoke marijuana I feel I can better cope with my emotions. My joints don't ache — in fact they feel better. My whole body seems to relax. I don't start to spasm, my neck doesn't hurt, my shoulders don't feel cramped. Just the opposite.

Finally, marijuana makes me feel like I'm in control. I smoke just enough marijuana to get the relief from nausea I need. When I feel my stomach unclench I stop smoking. It's simple. I've never run into any weird problems. I don't get to feeling out of control. My heartbeat might increase a little, but I don't feel like it's going to pop out of my chest.

I don't know why Marinol doesn't work as well as marijuana. But it just doesn't. Maybe some people who can't smoke will find Marinol helpful. I realize when I had PCP (*pneumocystis carinii pneumonia*) I couldn't smoke. I had trouble enough tying to breath. But when it came right down to a choice between taking Marinol or dealing with nausea, nausea won hands down. I can cope with being sick to my stomach. I don't like feeling out of my mind.

Shortly after I got out of the hospital I smoked marijuana again. It worked. Just like it has always worked. If I get PCP again I'm not taking Marinol. Instead, Kenny is going to make me some marijuana cookies.

Other PWAs have contacted the Alliance for Cannabis Therapeutics (ACT) and shared these thoughts about Marinol.

Comments of Tony Minarik of Tampa, Florida:

Marinol made me sick. I took 5 mg., like the *Physicians Desk Reference* said. It made me dizzy,

I felt very agitated and couldn't lie down or remain still. I just couldn't get comfortable. Marinol replaced the nausea with a pain in my stomach and I got a severe headache. I did manage to eat. But I was only eating to replace the pain in my stomach. With Marinol I didn't enjoy eating.

There's no similarity between Marinol and marijuana. Marinol was unpleasant, it made me feel worse, not better. Marinol and marijuana is the difference between night and day. With marijuana I smoke a few puffs and feel better. I'm hungry and actually enjoy eating when I smoke marijuana. My general outlook improves and my leg cramps go away.

Marinol is no substitute for marijuana.

It seems crazy to me that the government won't give me marijuana. My doctors routinely prescribe demerol, narcotics, all sorts of other dangerous drugs. They are perfectly willing to make me into a legal zombie. But they can't give me marijuana.

Comments of Rocky Laney, San Diego, California:

Marinol is ok sometimes. And sometimes Marinol fails to work and I feel very nauseated. Marijuana always works. Marijuana never fails to work.

When I wake up I'm often sick to my stomach. But when I'm gagging and throwing up Marinol just doesn't work. When I'm sick I can't wait for 30 to 60 minutes to get relief. And sometimes I throw the Marinol pill up. With marijuana I can just take one puff and the nausea melts away. Marijuana is instant relief. I don't need to wait around to get the relief I need.

Marijuana works quicker and it works better than Marinol.

Comments of Jeff Clay, Oceanside, California:

Marinol doesn't really seem to work. Marinol sometimes helps with the nausea, but it makes me feel stupid—like a zombie. On Marinol I've only gained 3 lbs. after two months of use. Marinol also seems less effective the longer I take it. I've taken Marinol and become disoriented. Several times I've started crying for no apparent reason. Marinol makes me real quiet. I get anxious, edgy. I don't want to be around people, I don't want to do anything, I don't want to go out. When I take Marinol I don't even answer the phone.

I like marijuana. Unlike Marinol, marijuana has an immediate effect, I don't have to wait for hours for relief. With marijuana relief is nearly instantaneous. My appetite is more stimulated by smoking, then when I take Marinol. I like being around people when I smoke, I like to laugh and have fun. It's very different than how I feel on Marinol.

If I had my choice I would choose marijuana, no question.

Comments of Daniel Parsons, Gonic, New Hampshire:

I've been taking Marinol for more than a year. But it's very hard to regulate. It doesn't stimulate my appetite. If I take two Marinol I fall asleep. I don't get any "high" from Marinol.

Marijuana triggers my appetite. Marijuana is a lot easier to control than the Marinol pill. I usually smoke about ¾ of a joint. If I smoke marijuana an hour before eating I can sit down and have a good dinner. When I have marijuana I eat three square meals a day.

After I was diagnosed with AIDS my weight went from 147 to 131 lbs. But when I smoke marijuana my weight increases. The real problem is being able to afford street marijuana.

Comments of Richard Cantwell, Philadelphia, Pennsylvania:

Marijuana doesn't make me want to cry.

Marinol makes me cry. Marinol makes me feel anguished. Marinol doesn't increase my appetite. Sometimes I burp after taking Marinol and it has a terrible, bitter taste. Marinol doesn't relieve my nausea, but it reduces my feeling I'm going to throw up. But the emotional turmoil, the sense of being overwhelmed makes Marinol a very unattractive product. Marinol is depressing.

Marinol also makes my eyes feel strange; I become very sensitive to light and my eyes feel strained. I don't like Marinol.

Marijuana soothes my stomach to the point where I actually enjoy eating. I smoke just before I eat—10 or 15 minutes. I can eat a full meal and I don't feel like I'm going to vomit half way through the meal. After I eat I don't throw up. Marijuana totally reduces my sense of anxiety. Unlike Marinol, marijuana relieves my anxiety it doesn't increase it.

I have Marinol available to me by prescription, but often won't use it because of the adverse mental and emotional effects it produces. I would never hesitate to smoke marijuana. They simply are not comparable products. The difference between Marinol and marijuana is profound. Marijuana actually works.

Comments of T.W., Sherman Oaks, California

It takes Marinol a long time to work— about an hour and a half. Marinol failed to help with my nausea and I didn't feel like eating. On Marinol I felt like I'd eaten marijuana brownies. Marinol made me feel spacey, it slowed me down, and I felt like I was under water. I was uncomfortable and I wanted it to stop. Marinol made me feel disconnected and apathetic. I stopped taking Marinol after these experiences.

With marijuana my nausea goes away in about 20 minutes. Then I get hungry and want to eat. I get the munchies and I eat everything in sight. When I smoke marijuana my weight increases because I eat so much more. Marijuana makes me feel comfortable with my surrounding, I enjoy thinking and I'm able to cope with my disease and deal with the problems in my life better. Marijuana allows me to view things more philosophically. If this sense of well being is euphoria, then marijuana makes me feel euphoric. What's so wrong with that?

Comments of Michael Newman, Orlando, Florida:

Marinol helped me calm down. But food-wise Marinol didn't help at all. Marinol helped reduce my nausea, but it did not help me eat. I don't like Marinol because it doesn't help me mentally or emotionally cope with my disease.

When I smoke marijuana it sets my mind to thinking about other things—things not connected with AIDS. Marijuana stops my nausea within about 15 minutes. Within a half hour to forty-five minutes I'm able to eat two to three times as much as usual. When I smoke marijuana I finish everything on my plate. Then I ask for seconds. Marijuana has increased my weight from 140 to 175 lbs. My lover can see a big difference when I smoke marijuana. I'm calmer, I eat better, my mood is better. When I smoke marijuana small things don't make me anxious or annoyed.

I recently told a friend of mine who was losing a lot of weight about smoking marijuana to help deal with AIDS. At first he was real skeptical, but then he watched me smoke and eat. Now he smokes marijuana. Since he started smoking he doesn't throw up anymore and his weight has stabilized.

I've been HIV+ since 1983. Without marijuana I know I would not be alive today. If I have a choice

between Marinol or marijuana I'd always choose
marijuana.

Open Forum Discussions of Marinol

The AIDS epidemic has spawned a large number of networking oppor-
tunities for individuals infected with HIV. These range from local support
groups to online, computer bulletin boards where individuals can con-
verse with others electronically.

The following items were retrieved from two online computer networks,
the Bay Area Bulletin Board Service based in San Francisco, California
and the National Association of People With AIDS (NAPWA) Link, in
Washington, D.C. (Further information can be found in Appendix C.)

The following comments have been retrieved from the Open Forum
sections of these online networks.

From: icon
Date: Sept. 6, 1990
Subject: Marinol

If there is anyone out there who knows anything about the drug Marinol, a
drug used to curb nausea so that PWAs with wasting syndrome can eat,
would you please leave me a message by E-Mail, Attn: Icon.

To: icon
Date: Sept. 26, 1990
Reply to item: Marinol

Marinol (Roxanne Laboratories, Columbus, Ohio, generic name dronabinol)
is synthetic marijuana (delta-9-THC). It has been used for nearly 10 years in
controlling nausea and increasing appetite in cancer chemotherapy patients.
There is no mention of the off-label use in patients with HIV disease in the
peer-reviewed literature. The most extensive article about this off-label use in
HIV patients appeared in the January 1989 issue of Critical Path AIDS Project
newsletter [2062 Lombard St., Philadelphia, PA 19146; (215) 545-2212]. The
article describes anecdotal use in Philadelphia and presumably elsewhere, in
which weight gains of 20 and even 30 lbs. have been seen. In combination
with Compazine, Marinol was seen in cancer patients to be even more effective, with little drug-induced "high." The use of Marinol (a controlled substance)
has gained widespread use in Philadelphia. Roxanne Laboratories says that
there is on-going research of this use, but no information has been published

or is forthcoming. An update was published in the July-August issue of Critical Path AIDS Project newsletter.

From: peabody
Date: Jan. 11, 1991
Subject: Re: Marinol

Marinol makes me mildly spacey. I believe I took 10mg. It's nothing like actually smoking. It's like pot without the fun. I understand that Marinol is only part of the chemical that makes up marijuana and not the whole thing. I was very hungry all day yesterday when I took it, but that could be from prednisone, another drug I'm on. Also I wasn't nauseous, but since I didn't get my third chemo, there was no reason for me to be.

The bottom line is that I don't think Marinol works. I'd love to see marijuana legalized. Besides giving me an enjoyable feeling, it calms my stomach down, relieves nausea, enables me to eat when otherwise I thought I couldn't.

From: peabody
To: alliance
Date: April 19, 1991
Subject: Re: Oasis at end of tunnel

I think you'd be interested in knowing that at this point in my medical sojourn, both my internist and oncologist unhesitatingly recommend pot for the nausea. This is the nausea that comes with the morphine (as opposed to chemotherapy nausea). The morphine does make me even more nauseous than the chemo did, — no vomiting, just waves of incredible dizzy nausea.

Why do they have to wait so long before giving patients the ultimate relief (morphine). There are plenty of PWAs with painful neuropathy but these stingy doctors wait for something like a lymphoma diagnosis before they can "justify" giving relief. It's a strange world.

From: peabody
Attn: alliance
Date: April 19, 1991
Subject: Re: Marinol

One of the advantages of pot over Marinol is that you get the benefit immediately after one toke. With Marinol you have to wait for it to be digested. And even then it's no where near as effective.

From: Spacecoast Surfer
To: MARS
Date: April 24, 1991

I never asked for the Marinol in the beginning because I didn't know that it was on the earth. The first prescription took over a week for the pills to get to Walgreen's from someplace in Memphis. Now the pharmacist has a supply. Very puzzling to me. I personally do not like the Marinol. I think it gives me too much of a buzz. So the black market is right around the corner. And I am forced to buy what works.

Conclusion

Should a person with HIV infection try Marinol for control of vomiting and appetite stimulation? The answer is almost always yes. Marinol is available by prescription and it does work for some patients. As with any drug—including marijuana—the patient and physician must work together to determine if Marinol can be effective. For some individuals Marinol can be an important "back-up" drug, providing relief when supplies of natural marijuana are not available.

For some patients Marinol is the solution. For others, as the above comments illustrate, it doesn't work at all or the side-effects are so severe that it simply cannot be tolerated.

In the war for drugs in the battle against AIDS, Marinol has a place in the physicians' armamentarium, just as marijuana does. It is not a question of which is best at the exclusion of the other, it is a question of providing every possible means of therapeutic relief, no matter the form or the politics. It is a matter of caring and a question of common sense.

IV. LEGAL ACCESS

Chapter Nine

MARIJUANA·AIDS RESEARCH SERVICE (MARS)

On the following pages is the protocol prepared by the Marijuana· AIDS Research Service. Individuals are encouraged to contact MARS (See Appendix C) for current information on compassionate access to marijuana and required application forms.

1571 front

DEPARTMENT OF HEALTH AND HUMAN SERVICES PUBLIC HEALTH SERVICE FOOD AND DRUG ADMINISTRATION **INVESTIGATIONAL NEW DRUG APPLICATION (IND)** *(TITLE 21, CODE OF FEDERAL REGULATIONS (CFR) Part 312)*	*Form Approved: OMB No. 0910-0014.* *Expiration Date: March 31, 1990.* *See OMB Statement on Reverse.* NOTE: No drug may be shipped or clinical investigation begun until an IND for that investigation is in effect (21 CFR 312.40).

1. NAME OF SPONSOR	2. DATE OF SUBMISSION

3. ADDRESS *(Number, Street, City, State and Zip Code)*	4. TELEPHONE NUMBER *(Include Area Code)*

5. NAME(S) OF DRUG *(Include all available names: Trade, Generic, Chemical, Code)* marijuana cigarettes, DEA code 7360	6. IND NUMBER *(If previously assigned)*

7. INDICATION(S) *(Covered by this submission)* Treatment of nausea and vomiting in HIV-positive individual. Also appetite stimulation. See attachment 12(6)(a).

8. PHASE (S) OF CLINICAL INVESTIGATION TO BE CONDUCTED: ☐ PHASE 1 ☐ PHASE 2 ☐ PHASE 3 ☐ OTHER _____ *(Specify)*

9. LIST NUMBERS OF ALL INVESTIGATIONAL NEW DRUG APPLICATIONS *(21 CFR Part 312)*, NEW DRUG OR ANTIBIOTIC APPLICATIONS *(21 CFR Part 314)*, DRUG MASTER FILES *(21 CFR 314.420)*, AND PRODUCT LICENSE APPLICATIONS *(21 CFR Part 601)* REFERRED TO IN THIS APPLICATION.

Reference NIDA master files 1631 and 366.

10. IND submissions should be consecutively numbered. The initial IND should be numbered *"Serial Number: 000."* The next submission (e.g., amendment, report, or correspondence) should be numbered *"Serial Number: 001."* Subsequent submissions should be numbered consecutively in the order in which they are submitted.	SERIAL NUMBER: – – –

11. THIS SUBMISSION CONTAINS THE FOLLOWING: *(Check all that apply)*

☒ INITIAL INVESTIGATIONAL NEW DRUG APPLICATION (IND)   ☐ RESPONSE TO CLINICAL HOLD

PROTOCOL AMENDMENT(S):   INFORMATION AMENDMENT(S):   IND SAFETY REPORT(S):

☐ NEW PROTOCOL   ☐ CHEMISTRY/MICROBIOLOGY   ☐ INITIAL WRITTEN REPORT
☐ CHANGE IN PROTOCOL   ☐ PHARMACOLOGY/TOXICOLOGY   ☐ FOLLOW-UP TO A WRITTEN REPORT
☐ NEW INVESTIGATOR   ☐ CLINICAL

☐ RESPONSE TO FDA REQUEST FOR INFORMATION   ☐ ANNUAL REPORT   ☐ GENERAL CORRESPONDENCE

☐ REQUEST FOR REINSTATEMENT OF IND THAT IS WITHDRAWN,   ☐ OTHER _____
INACTIVATED, TERMINATED OR DISCONTINUED   *(Specify)*

CHECK ONLY IF APPLICABLE

JUSTIFICATION STATEMENT MUST BE SUBMITTED WITH APPLICATION FOR ANY CHECKED BELOW. REFER TO THE CITED CFR SECTION FOR FURTHER INFORMATION.

☒ TREATMENT IND 21 CFR 312.35(b)   ☐ TREATMENT PROTOCOL 21 CFR 312.35(a)   ☐ CHARGE REQUEST/NOTIFICATION 21 CFR 312.7(d)

FOR FDA USE ONLY

CDR/DBIND/DGD RECEIPT STAMP	DDR RECEIPT STAMP	IND NUMBER ASSIGNED:
		DIVISION ASSIGNMENT:

FORM FDA 1571 (10/89)   PREVIOUS EDITION IS OBSOLETE.

1571 back

12. **CONTENTS OF APPLICATION**

This application contains the following items: *(check all that apply)*

☒ 1. Form FDA 1571 *[21 CFR 312.23 (a) (1)]*

☐ 2. Table of contents *[21 CFR 312.23 (a) (2)]*

☒ 3. Introductory statement *[21 CFR 312.23 (a) (3)]* See attachment 12(6)(a)

☒ 4. General investigational plan *[21 CFR 312.23 (a) (3)]* See attachment 12(6)(a)

☐ 5. Investigator's brochure *[21 CFR 312.23 (a) (5)]* See NIDA master files 1631 and 366.

6. Protocol(s) *[21 CFR 312.23 (a) (6)]*

    ☒ a. Study protocol(s) *[21 CFR 312.23 (a) (6)]*

    ☐ b. Investigator data *[21 CFR 312.23 (a) (6)(iii)(b)]* or completed Form(s) FDA 1572

    ☐ c. Facilities data *[21 CFR 312.23 (a) (6)(iii)(b)]* or completed Form(s) FDA 1572

    ☐ d. Institutional Review Board data *[21 CFR 312.23 (a) (6)(iii)(b)]* or completed Form(s) FDA 1572

☐ 7. Chemistry, manufacturing, and control data *[21 CFR 312.23 (a) (7)]* See NIDA master files 1631 and 366

    ☐ Environmental assessment or claim for exclusion *[21 CFR 312.23 (a) (7)(iv)(e)]*

☐ 8. Pharmacology and toxicology data *[21 CFR 312.23 (a) (8)]* See NIDA master files 1631 + 366

☐ 9. Previous human experience *[21 CFR 312.23 (a) (9)]* See NIDA master files 1631 + 366

☒ 10. Additional information *[21 CFR 312.23 (a) (10)]*

13. IS ANY PART OF THE CLINICAL STUDY TO BE CONDUCTED BY A CONTRACT RESEARCH ORGANIZATION? ☐ YES ☒ NO

IF YES, WILL ANY SPONSOR OBLIGATIONS BE TRANSFERRED TO THE CONTRACT RESEARCH ORGANIZATION? ☐ YES ☐ NO

IF YES, ATTACH A STATEMENT CONTAINING THE NAME AND ADDRESS OF THE CONTRACT RESEARCH ORGANIZATION, IDENTIFICATION OF THE CLINICAL STUDY, AND A LISTING OF THE OBLIGATIONS TRANSFERRED.

14. NAME AND TITLE OF THE PERSON RESPONSIBLE FOR MONITORING THE CONDUCT AND PROGRESS OF THE CLINICAL INVESTIGATIONS

15. NAME(S) AND TITLE(S) OF THE PERSON(S) RESPONSIBLE FOR REVIEW AND EVALUATION OF INFORMATION RELEVANT TO THE SAFETY OF THE DRUG

I agree not to begin clinical investigations until 30 days after FDA's receipt of the IND unless I receive earlier notification by FDA that the studies may begin. I also agree not to begin or continue clinical investigations covered by the IND if those studies are placed on clinical hold. I agree that an Institutional Review Board (IRB) that complies with the requirements set forth in 21 CFR Part 56 will be responsible for the initial and continuing review and approval of each of the studies in the proposed clinical investigation. I agree to conduct the investigation in accordance with all other applicable regulatory requirements.

16. NAME OF SPONSOR OR SPONSOR'S AUTHORIZED REPRESENTATIVE	**17.** SIGNATURE OF SPONSOR OR SPONSOR'S AUTHORIZED REPRESENTATIVE	
18. ADDRESS *(Number, Street, City, State and Zip Code)*	**19.** TELEPHONE NUMBER *(Include Area Code)*	**20.** DATE

(WARNING: A willfully false statement is a criminal offense. U.S.C. Title 18, Sec. 1001.)

Public reporting burden for this collection of information is estimated to average 30 minutes per response, including the time for reviewing instructions, searching existing data sources, gathering and maintaining the data needed, and completing reviewing the collection of information. Send comments regarding this burden estimate or any other aspect of this collection of information, including suggestions for reducing this burden to:

Reports Clearance Officer, PHS   and to: Office of Management and Budget
Hubert H. Humphrey Building, Room 721-H   Paperwork Reduction Project (0910-0014)
200 Independence Avenue, S.W.   Washington, DC 20503
Washington, DC 20201
Attn: PRA

*U.S.GPO:1989-261-200/08266

HIV/AIDS PROTOCOL

Investigator/Sponsor: _____, M.D.

Address: _____

_____

City:_____ State: _____ Zip _____

Phone: _____

Consulting: Robert Randall, Alliance for Cannabis Therapeutics, P.O. Box 21210, Kalorama Station, Washington, D.C. 20009; 202-483-8595

CONFIDENTIAL

The physician sponsoring this IND, and Mr. Robert Randall of the Alliance for Cannabis Therapeutics (ACT) are involved in making this submission. This application is strictly confidential. No information from this IND submission — or from the resulting reports — may be provided by the FDA to the DEA, NIDA, or to any group or individual, public or private, who is not directly involved in making this submission.

PURPOSE

The purpose of this study is to provide a seriously ill patient with licit, medically supervised access to marijuana for use in the reduction and control of emesis, anorexia, pain, and other symptoms caused by HIV infection.

This protocol encompasses a two year, single patient, compassionate IND. The physician reserves the right to request a continuation of this protocol beyond two years if the patient's condition warrants such extension.

JUSTIFICATION OF PURPOSE

Under this IND, access to marijuana is being requested for use in the treatment of an HIV-positive individual who is under therapy, and who is experiencing difficulty with conventional therapies. (See "Patient's Medical History Summary" below, for additional details.)

Patient's Medical History Summary

Patient's name: _____

Date of Birth: _____ **Sex:** _____ **Date of HIV diagnosis:**_____

1. Height & Weight:

Height: _____ft. _____ inches   Pre-diagnosis Weight: _____lbs.
Current Weight: _____lbs.   Total Weight Lost: _____lbs.

2. History of HIV-associated conditions (check all that apply):

☐ pneumocystis carinii pneumonia   ☐ Kaposi's Sarcoma   ☐ lymphoma
☐ anemia   ☐ toxoplasmosis   ☐ cryptosporidios   ☐ candida
☐ cryptococcal meningitis   ☐ mycobacterium avium intracellulare
☐ cytomegalovirus   ☐ Other (specify, use additional page if needed):

_____

3. Current Treatment(s) (check all that apply):

☐ AZT   ☐ DDI   ☐ Interferon   ☐ DDC   ☐ Bactrim   ☐ Pentamadine
☐ Antiemetic (please specify below)   ☐ Chemotherapy (specify below)
Antifungals: ☐ Clotrimazole   ☐ Flucorazole ☐ Ketoconazole   ☐ Nystatin
☐ Other (use additional page if necessary):_____

4. In addition to nausea, vomiting and weight loss does this patient also experience pain and/or spasms?   ☐ Yes   ☐ No

5. Has this patient smoked marijuana in the past?   ☐ Yes   ☐ No

6. Was marijuana helpful?   ☐ Yes   ☐ No

7. How was marijuana helpful? (check all that apply)

☐ Relieved nausea and/or vomiting   ☐ Stimulated appetite
☐ Reduced pain   ☐ Allowed a full night's sleep
☐ Reduced need for other medications   ☐ Eased muscle spasms
☐ Was better able to function

8. Additional comments and observations (use additional page if needed):

_____

Date   Physician's signature

BACKGROUND

There are numerous studies reported in historical and modern literature that demonstrate marijuana is useful in the treatment of emesis, the reduction of spasticity, and the control of chronic pain.

It is known that many HIV-infected patients do not respond well to conventional antiemetic, anti-spasmodic, and pain-control medicines. Employed in combination with powerful AIDS treatments such as AZT, extensive use of these pharmaceutical agents may provoke severe nausea and/or uncontrollable vomiting. Moreover, these drugs may also immobilize the patient and make it difficult for a person to function normally, perform simple tasks, or enjoy life.

It is also known that HIV-infection, as it advances, often causes a severe, even life-threatening loss of weight. PWAs, and persons with other HIV-related complications may lose 20% to 50% of their pre-diagnosis body weight. This drastic loss of weight can occur rapidly, further stressing the patient.

Currently available HIV-retarding therapies, like AZT, compound this disease-driven weight loss by subjecting the patient to drug-induced emesis. Even patients on the new, lower-dose regimen have difficultly tolerating protracted drug-induced emesis.

This combination of disease-driven anorexia and drug-induced emesis can be lethal. Such a condition places the patient at greater risk and greatly degrades the quality of life available to the patient. In despair, as many as half the patients receiving AZT therapy may be forced to discontinue treatment because of weight loss and emesis.

Evaluating marijuana's utility in easing the complications caused by HIV-infection and therapies could, therefore, provide physicians with insights into marijuana's role in treating the debilitating symptoms of AIDS and related conditions caused by HIV-infection.

Marijuana's well documented and extensively studied value as an antiemetic drug may benefit HIV-infected patients in the same way it provides relief to persons afflicted with various types of cancer who are undergoing emesis-provoking chemotherapy or radiation treatments.

Of similar import may be marijuana's often discussed utility as an appetite stimulant. Social smokers consistently report that marijuana enhances appetite. This effect is so pronounced and generally acknowledged it has worked its way into the common vocabulary as "the munchies."

If marijuana can ease emesis and induce hunger, then its therapeutic value to AIDS and other HIV-infected people may be considerable. The purpose of this protocol is to provide one such patient with licit access to this mode of therapy to evaluate the results.

Safety: There is a vast body of literature on marijuana's physical and psychological effects.[1] There is also highly specific information on marijuana's medical use in numerous therapeutic settings.[2]

In preparing this IND protocol the consultant reviewed medical reports and state studies with regard to marijuana's possible adverse effects. Based on these reports, past concerns over marijuana's safety for use under medical supervision have been greatly exaggerated.

- Reports from numerous investigators working in oncology, ophthalmology, and neurology, and from state authorized programs in New York, Michigan, New Mexico, Georgia, California, and Tennessee, indicate that marijuana, when smoked, is well tolerated by most patients, regardless of age. There were, in fact, surprisingly few serious adverse effects reported by these investigators. In no instance has any study found marijuana caused any patient severe biological injury or permanent mental distress. Given the range of drugs commonly employed in the treatment of HIV-infected persons, marijuana appears, by comparison, to be quite benign.

- Michigan evaluated patient acceptance and found cancer patients often preferred marijuana to more conventional antiemetic drugs.[3]

- Blood pressure changes: The only cautionary note concerns marijuana's potential affects on blood pressure as reported by Drs. John C. Merritt and William Crawford. Drs. Merritt and Crawford

---

1   Waller, Coy W. *et al.*, *Marijuana: An Annotated Bibliography, Macmillan Information:New York, 1976.*

2   Cohen, S. and Stillman, R.C. (eds.). *The Therapeutic Potential of Marijuana.* Plenum Publishing:New York, 1976). Also see: Mikuriya, Tod H. (ed.). *Marijuana Medical Papers.* Medi-Comp Press:Oakland, California, 1973.

3   Michigan Department of Public Health, 1983.

report a few patients given synthetic THC in oral form and marijuana may experience hypotension, a decline in blood pressure. Dr. Merritt encountered these problems when patients were compelled to smoke marijuana on a rigid time schedule.[4]

Significantly, several state programs report patients do much better when allowed to "self-titrate" rather than following a "standardized" smoking routine. After further investigation, Merritt noted that making simple alterations in the way patients smoked—most notably by permitting self-titration—completely eliminated this potential problem.

• Psychic distress appears to be rare among patients exposed to marijuana, but more common when synthetic THC (Marinol) is used.

• There has been some suggestion marijuana may function as an immunosuppressant. In reviewing the literature, however, research findings are at best contradictory.[5] Some studies actually suggest marijuana may enhance certain immune system responses. Significantly, Dr. J. Thomas Ungerleider of UCLA reports marijuana is an excellent anti-emetic drug for immunosuppressed patients afflicted with bone-marrow cancers. Indeed, Dr. Ungerleider indicates the use of a smokable antiemetic like marijuana is preferred over the use of oral antiemetics in such a situation.[6]

• Respiratory complications: evidence on marijuana's affect on pulmonary function is, at best, extremely incomplete. Clearly, marijuana may not be wise for patients suffering from severe respiratory complications like pneumonia. If this patient develops such difficulties, the use of marijuana will be discontinued until such

---

4   Merritt, John C., Crawford, William J., Alexander, Paul, Anduze, Alfred, L., & Gelbart, Solomon S. "Effect of Marijuana on Intraocular and Blood Pressure in Glaucoma." *Ophthalmology*, American Academy of Ophthalmology, Vol. 87, No. 3: pp. 222-228, March, 1980.

5   Hollister, Leo E. "Marijuana and Immunity." *Journal of Psychoactive Drugs*, 20(1): pp. 3-8, Jan-Mar. 1988.

6   R.C. Randall, (ed.). "Affidavit of J. Thomas Ungerleider, M.D." *Marijuana, Medicine & the Law, Vol. I*, Galen Press:Washington, D.C, 1988, p. 186.

time as its use may again be appropriate to the patient's medical needs.

- In evaluating marijuana's safety for use in the treatment of this patient it is important to remember that conventional therapies, while often ineffective in the treatment of HIV-infection or AIDS-induced emesis, anorexia, and weight loss are not without considerable risk. This is particularly true considering the powerful, highly addictive synthetic chemical substances that are required to provide even modest control over emesis, spasms, and chronic pain.

- Finally, it should be noted that after an extensive review of this question, DEA Administrative Law Judge Francis Young ruled marijuana is "safe for use under medical supervision" and determined efforts to argue marijuana is unsafe for medical use are "unreasonable, arbitrary, and capricious."

Given these conditions, and the gravity of the patient's prognosis, the physician believes marijuana can be safely employed in the treatment of HIV-related symptoms of emesis and weight loss.

Efficacy: Marijuana is being sought to treat several symptoms associated with this patient's condition. Primarily, marijuana is sought to control the debilitating emesis and weight loss this patient suffers as a consequence of continuing and intensive chemotherapy. Of equal interest is marijuana's appetite stimulant properties. Of secondary interest is marijuana's impact on pain and spasticity. Finally, there is the question of mental outlook. Does the use of marijuana alter this patient's emotional and intellectual perspectives? Do these alterations in perception improve the patient's ability to cope with this potentially terminal illness?

Emesis: Marijuana's utility as a safe, effective antiemetic is unchallenged. Studies by Sallan and Zinberg, NCI/Chang, and programs conducted by the states of New York, Michigan, New Mexico, Georgia, California, and Tennessee consistently demonstrate marijuana is highly effective and safe when employed to reduce emesis. Copies of reports from these studies and from the state-sponsored IND programs are available to—and on file with—the FDA. The fact all states report significant benefits and few adverse effects underscores the fact marijuana can be a highly effective antiemetic.[7]

In recent hearings before the DEA, the question of marijuana's use as an antiemetic was the subject of an extensive review. After taking testimony from many witnesses, the Court ruled to ignore marijuana's therapeutic use in the reduction of emesis is "arbitrary, capricious, and irrational."[7]

Appetite Stimulant: Evidence on marijuana's utility as an appetite stimulant seems less certain. Unfortunately, much of this work has been conducted on psychologically anorexic patients who, generally, do not want to eat. However, reports from patients, and from participating physicians in the state programs strongly suggest marijuana is an effective appetite stimulant. In New Mexico, for example, the FDA approved continuing use of marijuana by one patient specifically for purposes of appetite stimulation.

Pain & Spasms: It has been demonstrated by Dunn and Davis[8] and Petro and Ellenberger[9] that marijuana can significantly reduce spasticity. These studies were prompted by anecdotal accounts from spasticity patients concerning their use of marijuana and its beneficial effects on their conditions.

Historical accounts of marijuana's use in the treatment of pain and spasticity are extensive, particularly in the medical literature of the late 19th Century. For example, as early as March 22, 1890, Dr. J. Russell Reynolds writes, "There are many cases of so-called epilepsy in adults, but which, in my opinion, (are) the result of organic disease of a gross character in the nervous centers, in which India hemp [marijuana] is the most useful agent with which I am acquainted."

In recent hearings before the DEA, the question of marijuana's use in the reduction of spasm and the treatment of chronic pain were the subject of an extensive review. After taking testimony from many witnesses, the Court ruled that to ignore marijuana's therapeutic use in the reduction of spasms and in the treatment of chronic pain is "arbitrary, capricious, and irrational."[10]

---

7   Decision of Judge Francis L. Young. *Marijuana, Medicine & The Law, Volume II.* Galen Press:Washington, D.C., 1989, pp. 407-446.

8   Dunn, M. and Davis, Floyd. "The Perceived Effects of Marijuana on Spinal Cord Injured Males." *Paraplegia,* 12(3):p. 175, 1974.

9   Petro, Denis and Ellenberger, Carl. "Marijuana May Lessen Spasticity of MS." *JAMA* Vol. 241, No. 23:p. 2476, June 9, 1979.

PROCEDURES

This protocol will evaluate marijuana's utility in controlling or reducing the symptoms associated with HIV-infection. The patient has a well documented medical history. This will make extensive pre-evaluations unnecessary as the patient's history provides an ample "baseline" point of departure.

Immediately prior to initiation of marijuana therapy, however, the patient will be given a standard physical examination to establish baseline data for later comparison. This data will include the patient's weight.

On several occasions during the first month of treatment with marijuana, the patient will report to the physician. During these sessions we will review the situation. This procedure will be repeated several times during the first few months of treatment.

If these evaluations indicate marijuana significantly reduces the patient's emesis, chronic pain, and/or muscle spasms, and there is no evidence of serious adverse effects, the patient may elect to continue treatment. If the patient elects to continue with this mode of treatment they will be seen by the physician at least once monthly.

The physician will work with the patient to establish a viable therapeutic dose that effectively reduces symptoms without causing any untoward side effects.

If, at the conclusion of the first month of treatment an effective therapeutic dose can be established, there is no evidence of serious adverse effects, and the patient appears to be responding well they will be placed on long-term care using marijuana.

Once placed on continuing care the patient will be seen by the physician once monthly. During these meetings the physician will record the patient's weight, determine if any noticeable change has occurred in the patient's condition, and, if all is stable, issue another prescription for marijuana to the patient.

---

10   Decision of Judge Francis L. Young. *In The Matter Of Marijuana Rescheduling.* DEA:Washington, D.C., September 6, 1988.

At approximately six-month intervals, the physician will conduct a basic physical examination and discuss marijuana's effects with the patient. A number of factors will be used by the physician in determining outcome.

- Weight stabilization or gain would suggest improved appetite and increased caloric intake.

- A decline in the patient's use of prescription drugs (particularly pain-killing drugs and antiemetics) would suggest improved control over symptoms.

- Ability to function and cope with the infection will be assessed through conversation and physical examination.

The information collected during these six-month reviews, and the briefer information collected on a monthly basis, will allow the physician to reach certain conclusions about marijuana's proper role in the treatment of HIV-infected persons. These conclusions will be reported to FDA, as described below.

DRUG SUPPLY

This protocol will employ marijuana as provided in pre-rolled cigarette form (DEA Code #7360) by the NIDA . These NIDA provided cigarettes should be of at least 2% THC content or higher. Several studies strongly suggest the reduction in emesis, pain relief, reduction of spasticity, and diminution of his other symptoms appear to be dose related. Therefore, cigarettes of less than 2% THC content may not be adequate to this patient's therapeutic needs.

OTHER DRUGS TO BE USED

The patient may, during the course of therapy, employ a large number of drugs to control infection, ease pain, and reduce spasticity and other HIV-infection symptoms. Under this protocol the patient will continue using these other drugs during the initial stages of marijuana therapy. Any alteration in this patient's present drug therapy will only be undertaken if symptoms are well controlled or to prevent the development of serious adverse effects.

The patient's need for prescriptive pain killing and mood altering drugs, such as benzodiazepines or Marinol will provide one objective means of determining how effectively marijuana is controlling chronic pain. If this patient's need for these substances is significantly reduced, this objective measure will provide one means of determining how effective marijuana is as a pain management agent.

INFORMED CONSENT

The patient is mentally competent and has given written, informed consent to participate in this compassionate IND evaluation. The potential side effects of marijuana use have been explained in detail. There appear to be no serious medical contraindications to this patient's use of marijuana within a supervised routine of medical care.

DISPENSING THE DRUG

The marijuana used in this study will be provided to the patient through a pharmacy located near the patient's home or through one of the several hospital/clinic pharmacies serving HIV patients in the area. The precise pharmacy to be selected will be one agreeable to the physician and patient. This pharmacy should be accessible to the patient.

The pharmacy favored by the physician and patient is:

Pharmacy name: _____

Hospital/Clinic: _____

Street address: _____

City: _____ State: _____ Zip: _____

Telephone: _____

REPORTS

The sponsor will provide the FDA with yearly reports on this patient's progress. These reports will include information on the patient's present medical status and use of marijuana.

The sponsor will report any serious marijuana-induced, life-threatening adverse effects to the FDA within 72 hours, and the physician will immediately discontinue the patient's access to marijuana until the nature of the effect and its consequences can be properly evaluated.

PATIENT CONSENT FORM

I, _____, understand that
this study will evaluate marijuana's use in the treatment of symptoms
of HIV-infection or AIDS with special focus on nausea and vomiting,
weight loss, chronic pain and muscle spasticity caused by severe HIV-
infection and/or HIV-retarding therapies. As a patient who suffers from
HIV-infection and experiences severe nausea and/or vomiting, intense
pain and/or muscle spasticity, I am interested in marijuana's potential
medical uses and I volunteer to participate in this study of marijuana's
effect on my above mentioned symptoms.

I realize in addition to marijuana's possible benefits in controlling
nausea and vomiting, easing pain and reducing spasticity, the drug may
also cause various side effects including, but not limited to, alterations
in consciousness and mood, anxiety, euphoria, drowsiness, depression,
disorientation, paranoia, confusion, rapid pulse, pounding of the heart,
dizziness, fainting, bloodshot eyes, and dryness of the mouth. Although
not validated by clinical studies, I understand some researchers believe
marijuana may cause damage to the lungs and brain, changes in
hormone levels, personality changes and other psychological problems.
However, I also understand marijuana, at the dosages I am to receive,
has been well tolerated by other patients who smoke marijuana to reduce
intraocular pressures, control nausea and vomiting and ease spasticity.
Due to marijuana's reported intoxicating side effects I agree not to operate
a car or other motor vehicle if I become intoxicated while smoking
marijuana.

During this study I will be under the care of my doctor. If I leave my
doctor's care I understand my access to marijuana will be terminated
unless another physician responsible for my care receives FDA approval
to provide me with marijuana. I also understand that if for any reason I
decide to leave this program, my doctor will notify the FDA of my decision
and marijuana will be unavailable to me for this purpose.

Signed _____ Date_____

Witness _____ Date_____

Witness _____ Date_____

FDA Form #1571 Section 12 (10)

Additional Attachments

A. The Consent Form to be employed for this study is a standard Consent Form employed in similar programs.

B. The sponsor will notify the U.S. Food & Drug Administration (FDA) if this program is discontinued. Such notification will include a statement of reasons for the program's discontinuation.

C. Marijuana cigarettes used in this program will be provided to the patient without cost.

D. The sponsor will submit a copy of the treatment plan (attachment #12(6)(a) to FD Form #1571) and Patient Informed Consent Form to an Institutional Review Board (IRB) and will not proceed with the compassionate IND until it has been reviewed and approved by the IRB.

_____

Physician's signature

_____

Date

1572 form

DEPARTMENT OF HEALTH AND HUMAN SERVICES PUBLIC HEALTH SERVICE FOOD AND DRUG ADMINISTRATION **STATEMENT OF INVESTIGATOR** *(TITLE 21, CODE OF FEDERAL REGULATIONS (CFR) Part 312)* (See instructions on reverse side.)	Form Approved: OMB No. 0910-0014 Expiration Date: November 30, 1989 *See OMB Statement on Reverse.*
	NOTE: No investigator may participate in an investigation until he/she provides the sponsor with a completed, signed Statement of Investigator, Form FDA 1572 (21 CFR 312.53(c))

1. NAME AND ADDRESS OF INVESTIGATOR.

2. EDUCATION, TRAINING, AND EXPERIENCE THAT QUALIFIES THE INVESTIGATOR AS AN EXPERT IN THE CLINICAL INVESTIGATION OF THE DRUG FOR THE USE UNDER INVESTIGATION. ONE OF THE FOLLOWING IS ATTACHED:

☐ CURRICULUM VITAE   ☐ OTHER STATEMENT OF QUALIFICATIONS

3. NAME AND ADDRESS OF ANY MEDICAL SCHOOL, HOSPITAL, OR OTHER RESEARCH FACILITY WHERE THE CLINICAL INVESTIGATION(S) WILL BE CONDUCTED.

4. NAME AND ADDRESS OF ANY CLINICAL LABORATORY FACILITIES TO BE USED IN THE STUDY.

5. NAME AND ADDRESS OF THE INSTITUTIONAL REVIEW BOARD (IRB) THAT IS RESPONSIBLE FOR REVIEW AND APPROVAL OF THE STUDY(IES).

6. NAMES OF THE SUBINVESTIGATORS (*e.g., research fellows, residents, associates*) WHO WILL BE ASSISTING THE INVESTIGATOR IN THE CONDUCT OF THE INVESTIGATION(S).

7. NAME AND CODE NUMBER, IF ANY, OF THE PROTOCOL(S) IN THE IND FOR THE STUDY(IES) TO BE CONDUCTED BY THE INVESTIGATOR.

FORM FDA 1572 (8/89)   PREVIOUS EDITION IS OBSOLETE.

1572 form

8. ATTACH THE FOLLOWING CLINICAL PROTOCOL INFORMATION:

☐ FOR PHASE 1 INVESTIGATIONS, A GENERAL OUTLINE OF THE PLANNED INVESTIGATION INCLUDING THE ESTIMATED DURATION OF THE STUDY AND THE MAXIMUM NUMBER OF SUBJECTS THAT WILL BE INVOLVED.

☐ FOR PHASE 2 OR 3 INVESTIGATIONS, AN OUTLINE OF THE STUDY PROTOCOL INCLUDING AN APPROXIMATION OF THE NUMBER OF SUBJECTS TO BE TREATED WITH THE DRUG AND THE NUMBER TO BE EMPLOYED AS CONTROLS, IF ANY; THE CLINICAL USES TO BE INVESTIGATED; CHARACTERISTICS OF SUBJECTS BY AGE, SEX, AND CONDITION; THE KIND OF CLINICAL OBSERVATIONS AND LABORATORY TESTS TO BE CONDUCTED; THE ESTIMATED DURATION OF THE STUDY; AND COPIES OR A DESCRIPTION OF CASE REPORT FORMS TO BE USED.

9. COMMITMENTS:

I agree to conduct the study(ies) in accordance with the relevant, current protocol(s) and will only make changes in a protocol after notifying the sponsor, except when necessary to protect the safety, rights, or welfare of subjects.

I agree to personally conduct or supervise the described investigation(s).

I agree to inform any patients, or any persons used as controls, that the drugs are being used for investigational purposes and I will ensure that the requirements relating to obtaining informed consent in 21 CFR Part 50 and institutional review board (IRB) review and approval in 21 CFR Part 56 are met.

I agree to report to the sponsor adverse experiences that occur in the course of the investigation(s) in accordance with 21 CFR 312.64.

I have read and understand the information in the investigator's brochure, including the potential risks and side effects of the drug.

I agree to ensure that all associates, colleagues, and employees assisting in the conduct of the study(ies) are informed about their obligations in meeting the above commitments.

I agree to maintain adequate and accurate records in accordance with 21 CFR 312.62 and to make those records available for inspection in accordance with 21 CFR 312.68.

I will ensure that an IRB that complies with the requirements of 21 CFR Part 56 will be responsible for the initial and continuing review and approval of the clinical investigation. I also agree to promptly report to the IRB all changes in the research activity and all unanticipated problems involving risks to human subjects or others. Additionally, I will not make any changes in the research without IRB approval, except where necessary to eliminate apparent immediate hazards to human subjects.

I agree to comply with all other requirements regarding the obligations of clinical investigators and all other pertinent requirements in 21 CFR Part 312.

INSTRUCTIONS FOR COMPLETING FORM FDA 1572
STATEMENT OF INVESTIGATOR:

1. Complete all sections. Attach a separate page if additional space is needed.

2. Attach curriculum vitae or other statement of qualifications as described in Section 2.

3. Attach protocol outline as described in Section 8.

4. Sign and date below.

5. FORWARD THE COMPLETED FORM AND ATTACHMENTS TO THE SPONSOR. The sponsor will incorporate this information along with other technical data into an Investigational New Drug Application (IND). INVESTIGATORS SHOULD NOT SEND THIS FORM DIRECTLY TO THE FOOD AND DRUG ADMINISTRATION.

10. SIGNATURE OF INVESTIGATOR

11 DATE

Public reporting burden for this collection of information is estimated to average 1 hour per response, including the time for reviewing instructions, searching existing data sources, gathering and maintaining the data needed, and completing reviewing the collection of information. Send comments regarding this burden estimate or any other aspect of this collection of information, including suggestions for reducing this burden to:

Reports Clearance Officer, PHS   and to: Office of Management and Budget
Hubert H. Humphrey Building, Room 721-H   Paperwork Reduction Project (0910-0014)
200 Independence Avenue, S.W.   Washington, DC 20503
Washington, DC 20201
Attn: PRA

FORM FDA 1572 (8/89)   *U.S. Government Printing Office: 1989-241-264/08260

Chapter Ten

COMMONLY ASKED QUESTIONS*

Is marijuana available by prescription?

No. Marijuana is classified by the federal government as a Schedule I drug and is not available by prescription.

Can marijuana be obtained legally for medical purposes?

Yes. Physicians who wish to treat HIV-positive patients with marijuana may file a compassionate investigational new drug (IND) application with the Food and Drug Administration (FDA).

Does marijuana help HIV-positive patients?

Yes. Studies conducted in the 1970s and 1980s show marijuana is one of the most effective anti-nausea and vomiting drugs known to man. Marijuana also improves appetite. Many HIV patients and people with AIDS (PWAs) experience nausea and vomiting as a result of AZT or other drugs. Additionall,y the "wasting syndrome" is a serious problem for HIV and AIDS patients. Marijuana helps the patient maintain body weight and this, in turn, helps the patient fight infections.

Are these just patient "impressions?"

No. Studies show marijuana reduces the nausea and vomiting caused by many toxic drugs. Studies on cancer patients permitted to legally smoke marijuana in New Mexico, California, Michigan, New York, Georgia, and Tennessee reveal marijuana often reduces nausea and vomiting even when all available prescription drugs fail to work.

---

*   Originally prepared by the Alliance for Cannabis Therapeutics and the Marijuana•AIDS Research Service (MARS).

Does marijuana harm the immune system?

No. More than 35 studies have evaluated marijuana's effects on the immune system. Based on these studies the highly respected *Journal of Psychoactive Drugs* determined marijuana has no significant effect—negative or positive—on the immune system. According to the *Journal*, studies purporting to show harm to the immune system by marijuana "have been seriously flawed" by using high concentrations of synthetic delta-9-THC and have been conducted in test tubes and cultures, not in humans. Highly toxic drugs like AZT have a far more damaging effect on the immune system than marijuana.

Is marijuana safe?

Yes. The chief administrative law judge of the Drug Enforcement Administration (DEA) recently ruled, "Marijuana is one of the safest therapeutically active substances known to man." He also concluded marijuana is "capable of relieving the distress of great numbers of very ill people, and doing so with safety under medical supervision." HIV-positive people who contact the Alliance for Cannabis Therapeutics (ACT) report marijuana is safe. They have decided marijuana's few negative effects (*e.g.*, sleepiness, red-eyes, dry-mouth) are more than off-set by the drug's powerful anti-nausea and appetite stimulating properties. These people report marijuana dramatically improves the quality of life and helps stabilize weight. Many report a weight gain after they begin smoking marijuana. PWAs who have used marijuana medically report the drug allows a "more normal life" with relatively few side-effects.

Is there a "pot pill"?

Yes. Marinol is synthetic THC, the chemical in marijuana that causes the "high." Marinol is available by prescription, but PWAs consistently report the synthetic drug is far less effective than natural marijuana. Studies on cancer chemotherapy patients also show the THC/Marinol "pot pill" is less effective than smoked marijuana. Marinol is also more likely to cause side effects.

Does my doctor need to apply to any federal agencies other than the FDA?

Yes. Your doctor must also file Form #225 with the Drug Enforcement Administration (DEA). All doctors have received a DEA registration number in order to prescribe other drugs, but they must register separately in order to obtain marijuana.

Who supplies the marijuana?

The DEA provides special order forms for marijuana that must be sent to the National Institute on Drug Abuse (NIDA). The NIDA will ship marijuana to the designated pharmacy.

Where does the NIDA obtain the marijuana?

The NIDA grows and harvests marijuana at the University of Mississippi. The harvested marijuana is shipped to North Carolina where it is dose qualified and rolled into cigarettes.

When will we hear from the FDA?

By law the FDA must respond to an IND application within 30 days. There is no statutory requirement for the DEA to respond and the Agency usually requires repeated prodding. Doctors are urged to keep copies of all correspondence with federal agencies and to mail all items "return receipt requested."

Does the DEA have a right to reject the physician's compassionate IND request?

No. The DEA's only function is to check the "security" of the drug.

What does that mean?

After an IND is approved marijuana must be shipped from North Carolina to the appropriate pharmacy. Storage is required on the receiving end and this is where the DEA gets involved. Sometimes the DEA will attempt to "persuade" the doctor to store marijuana in his or her office. The Alliance strongly recommends against this practice. It places the doctor in the awkward position of acting as a pharmacist.

Where should the marijuana be stored?

The marijuana should be stored at a pharmacy just like other medically useful drugs. All reputable pharmacies already comply with stringent DEA regulations for drug security. Furthermore, a pharmacy is better equipped to re-order the drug as needed.

Can this be a corner pharmacy?

Perhaps. In most cases the DEA insists on a hospital pharmacy but there has been at least one case in which a "corner drugstore" was authorized to store and dispense marijuana. Security is the most important element. Veterans are encouraged to consider a VA hospital pharmacy.

Hasn't the federal government tried to stop compassionate access to marijuana?

Yes. Efforts have been made to terminate the compassionate IND program. To date these efforts have been unsuccessful. Patients desiring prescriptive access to marijuana are urged to contact the Alliance for current information on the status of the compassionate IND program.

All of this sounds very complicated. Can marijuana really be obtained legally?

Yes. But it takes the combined efforts of patient and physician. It also takes time and persistence.

V. APPENDICES

Appendix A

JENKS vs. FLORIDA

Opinion of the District Court of Appeal,
First District, State of Florida
April 16, 1991

Justice J. Ervin, for the Court

Kenneth and Barbra Jenks appeal their convictions for cultivation of marijuana and possession of drug paraphernalia, contending that the trial court erred in refusing to recognize their defense of medical necessity. We agree and reverse.

Kenneth Jenks inherited hemophilia from his mother, and contracted the acquired immune deficiency syndrome (AIDS) virus from a blood transfusion. He unknowingly passed it to his wife, Barbra Jenks. Mrs. Jenks' health began to decline rapidly. Her weight dropped from 150 to 112 lbs. during a 3 week period as a result of constant vomiting, and she was hospitalized at least 6 times for 2 to 3 weeks at a time. Although she had been prescribed over a half-dozen oral medications for nausea, none of them worked. When given shots for nausea, she was left in a stupor and unable to function. Likewise, when Mr. Jenks started AZT treatment he was not able to eat because the medication left him constantly nauseous. He also lost weight, although not as dramatically as his wife.

When the Jenks began participating in a support group sponsored by the Bay County Health Department, a group member told them how marijuana had helped him. Although initially reluctant, Mr. and

139

Mrs. Jenks tried marijuana and found that they were able to retain their AIDS medications, eat, gain weight, maintain their health, and stay out of the hospital. They asked their treating physician about prescribing the drug, but were unable to obtain a legal prescription.[1] The Jenks decided to grow two marijuana plants to insure its availability, avoid the expense of buying it on the street, and reduce the possibility of arrest.

On March 29, 1990, the Jenks were arrested and charged with manufacturing (cultivating) cannabis, pursuant to Section 893.13, Florida Statutes (1989), and possession of drug paraphernalia, a violation of Section 893.147, Florida Statutes (1989). The Jenks admitted to cultivating the marijuana and advised officers at the scene that they each had AIDS and used the marijuana to relieve their symptoms.

The Jenks waived their right to a jury trial and agreed that the bench trial should center on their defense of medical necessity. Because their physician, Dr. Thomas Sunnenberg, was not available to testify, the parties agreed to the following pretrial stipulation:

> Defense witness, Thomas D. Sunnenberg, M.D. ... will testify as follows:
>
> 8. That he has been unable to find any effective drug for treating the defendants' nausea.
>
> 9. That the nausea is so debilitating that if it is not controlled, the defendants could die.
>
> 10. That if he could legally prescribe *cannabis sativa* as a drug to control their nausea he would.
>
> 11. That the only drug that controls their nausea is *cannabis sativa.*
>
> 12. That he is presently seeking access to legal *cannabis sativa* through the Food and Drug Administration (FDA) under the compassionate investigational new drug program (IND) for the Jenks.

---

1   During the pendency of this appeal, the Jenks obtained permission from the federal government to use marijuana for control of nausea, vomiting, and weight loss caused by AIDS.

At trial, the defense also presented two expert witnesses, Robert Randall, who suffers from glaucoma and who successfully asserted the defense of medical necessity against a charge of marijuana cultivation in 1976,[2] and Dr. Daniel Dansak of Alabama, who has treated over 50 patients who have used marijuana to alleviate both disease symptoms and side-effects of medication.

The trial judge rejected the defense of medical necessity, found the Jenks guilty of manufacturing marijuana, and withheld adjudication of guilt, placing the Jenks on 1 year of unsupervised probation. He ordered the Jenks to perform 500 hours of community service, to be discharged only by "providing care, comfort, and concern for each other."

The necessity defense has been formulated as follows:

> The pressure of natural physical forces sometimes confronts a person in an emergency with a choice of two evils: either he may violate the literal terms of the criminal law and thus produce a harmful result, or he may comply with those terms and thus produce a greater or equal or lesser amount of harm. For reasons of social policy, if the harm which will result from compliances with the law is greater than that which will result from violation of it, he is by virtue of the defense of necessity justified in violating it.[3]

Although there is no specific legislative acceptance of the necessity defense in Florida, we conclude that the defense was recognized as common law and that there has been no clearly expressed legislative rejection of such defense. The necessity defense was articulated as early as 1551 in *Reninger v. Fagossa*, 1 Plowd. 1, 19, 75 Eng. Rep. 1, 29-30 (1551): "[W]here the words of [the law] are broken to avoid greater inconvenience, or through necessity, or by compulsion," the law has not been broken.[4] The authors state that the defense is poorly

---

2   United States v. Randall, 104 Daily Wash. L. Rep. 2249 (Super. Ct. D.C. Nov. 24, 1976).

3   W.R. LaFave v. A.W. Scott, Jr., 1 *Substantive Criminal Law* § 5.4, at 627 (1986) (hereinafter LaFave & Scott). Or, as stated by Justice Holmes, "Detached reflection cannot be expected in the presence of an uplifted knife." Arnolds & Garland, "The Defense of Necessity in Criminal Law: The Right to Choose the Lesser Evil," *J. Crim. L. & Criminology*, 65:289-290, (1974) (hereinafter Arnolds & Garland) [quoting *Brown v. United States*, 256 U.S. 335, 41 S.Ct. 501, 65 L.Ed. 961 (1921)].

developed in Anglo-American jurisprudence because there are so few cases dealing with it, "probably because these cases are not often prosecuted." In any event, they indicate that although there is some disagreement on this, "it seems clear that necessity was a defense at common law."[5] The authors cite a number of pre-1776 cases involving the necessity defense.[6]

Consequently, we consider that Florida has adopted the necessity defense pursuant to Section 2.01, Florida Statutes (1989), which provides:

> The common and statute laws of England which are of a general and not a local nature...are declared to be of force in this state; provided, the said statutes and common law be not inconsistent with the Constitution and laws of the United States and the acts of the Legislature of this state.

The medical-necessity defense is merely a more particular application of the necessity defense. See, *e.g.*, LaFave & Scott at §5.4(c)7, at 631-33; C.E. Torcia, 1 *Wharton's Criminal Law* §88 (1978); 22 C.J.S. *Criminal Law* §50 (1989). In fact, in *Bavero v. State*, 347 So.2d 781 (Fla. 1st DCA 1977), this Court recognized the defense of medical necessity there asserted by a prison escapee. *Accord State v. Alcantaro*, 407 So.2d 922, 924 (Fla. 1st DCA 1981) ("Medical necessity was recognized as an arguable defense by this Court in *Bavero v. State*[.]")., review denied, 413 So.2d 875 (Fla. 1982).

Although the state conceded at oral argument that the necessity defense exists in Florida's common law, the state nevertheless contends that Section 893.03, Florida Statutes (1989), is inconsistent with and therefore precludes the defense in the case at bar. We disagree. Section 893.03(1) provides:

> Schedule I.—A substance in Schedule I has a high potential for abuse and has no currently accepted medical use in treatment in the United States and in its use under medical supervision does not meet accepted safety standards except for such uses provided for in s.402.36. The following substances are controlled in Schedule I:

---

4   Arnolds & Garland, at 291.

5   Arnolds & Garland, at 290.

6   Arnolds & Garland, at 291 n.29. Other pre-1776 cases are cited in Note, "Necessity: The Right to Present a Recognized Defense," *N. Eng. L. Rev.*, 21:779, 781-83, 1985-86.

* * *

(c)4. Cannabis.

(Footnote omitted.) However, subsection (1)(d) provides,

> Notwithstanding the aforementioned fact that Schedule I substances have no currently accepted medical use, the Legislature recognizes that certain substances are currently accepted for certain limited medical uses in treatment in the United States but have a high potential for abuse.

The state argues that section 893.03 permits no medical uses of marijuana whatsoever. In fact, all that subsection (1) states is that marijuana is not generally available for medical use. Subsection (1)(d), however, clearly indicates that Schedule I substances may be subject to limited medical uses. It is well established that a statute should not be construed as abrogating the common law unless it speaks unequivocally, and should not be interpreted to displace common law more than is necessary. *Carlile v. Game & Fresh Water Fish Comm'n*, 354 So.2d 362, 364 (Fla. 1977) (quoting 30 Fla. Jur. *Statutes* §130 (rev. ed. 1974); *State v. Egan*, 287 So.2d 1, 6-7 (Fla. 1973); *Sullivan v. Leatherman*, 48 So.2d 836, 838 (Fla. 1950) (en banc). We conclude that section 893.03 does not preclude the defense of medical necessity under the particular facts of this case.

Moreover, we conclude that the Jenks met their burden of establishing this defense at trial. The elements of the defense have previously been addressed by trial courts in *United States v. Randall*, 104 Daily Wash. L. Rep. 2249 (Super. Ct. D.C. Nov. 24, 1976), and in Florida in *State v. Mussika*, 14 F.L.W. 1 (Fla. 17th Cir. Ct. Dec. 28, 1988), cases that involved the medically necessary use of marijuana by people with glaucoma. Those elements are as follows: 1) that the defendant did not intentionally bring about the circumstance which precipitated the unlawful act; 2) that the defendant could not accomplish the same objective using a less offensive alternative available to the defendant; and 3) that the evil sought to be avoided was more heinous than the unlawful act perpetuated to avoid it.

As applied to the case at bar, the Jenks obviously did not intend to contract AIDS. Furthermore, the parties stipulated that the Jenks' physician was unable to find an alternative drug that effectively eliminated or diminished his patients' nausea. Finally, the parties further stipulated that if the nausea was not controlled, the Jenks' lives were in danger. Based upon these facts, we conclude the trial court erred in rejecting the Jenks' defense and in convicting them as charged.

Reversed with directions that judgment of acquittal be entered.

Mehmer, J., concurs. Nimmons, J., dissents without written opinion.

Appendix B

AIDS CHRONOLOGY*

1981   **The first cases and first response**

June 5   The Centers for Disease Control (CDC) report the
              first cases of illness that will be known as AIDS.

July 3   A *New York Times* article announces a "Rare Can-
              cer Seen in 41 Homosexuals."

August 11   The first meeting of the group to become the Gay
              Men's Health Crisis (GMHC) is held.

October   The CDC categorizes the mysterious disease as an
              epidemic.

December 31   152 cases of the deadly new disease have been
              reported in the U.S.

1982   **The illness is named**

•   The disease, known as Gay-Related Immune
              Deficiency (GRID), Kaposi's Sarcoma, and "gay can-
              cer" is officially named acquired immune deficien-
              cy syndrome — AIDS.

•   The first federal funds — $5.6 million — are allo-
              cated to AIDS research.

Dec. 31   1,300 cases of AIDS have been reported in the
              U.S.; 317 are dead.

---

*   Originally prepared by the Gay Men's Health Crisis. Updated by the San
Francisco Aids Foundation and the Marijuana/AIDS Research Service.

1983   **The first challenge to discrimination**

•   The first AIDS discrimination suit, Sonnabend &
                Callen v. 49 W. 12th, is litigated by Lambda Legal
                Defense Fund and funded by GMHC. The suit is
                decided in favor of the plaintiffs.

Dec. 31   4,156 cases of AIDS have been reported in the
                U.S.; 1,292 are dead.

1984   **The cause of AIDS is identified**

•   Scientists prove conclusively that they have iso-
                lated the infectious agent believed to cause AIDS—
                now known has Human Immunodeficiency Virus
                (HIV).

Dec. 31   9,920 cases of AIDS have been reported in the
                U.S.; 3,665 are dead.

1985   **The new American ABC's: AIDS, Blood, Condoms**

March   The HIV antibody test is licensed. Screening of the
                blood supply begins. Condom use is shown to be
                effective in preventing sexual transmission of HIV.

July   Rock Hudson dies of AIDS.

•   AIDS cases have now been reported in every popu-
                lated continent in the world.

•   The first International Conference on AIDS is held.

Dec. 31   20,470 cases of AIDS have been reported in the
                U.S.; 8,161 are dead.

1986   **Condoms and confidentiality**

May   Surgeon General C. Everett Koop releases his
                report calling for AIDS education for children of all
                ages, and urging widespread use of condoms.

•   The AIDS Clinical Trial Groups are formed with
                $47 million from Congress.

Dec. 31   37,061 AIDS cases have been reported in the U.S.;
                16,301 people are dead.

1987　　　**ACT UP, AZT, and Jesse Helms**

Feb.

The AIDS Coalition to Unleash Power (ACT UP) is founded to end the AIDS crisis through direct action. The first action takes place on Wall Street.

March

AZT—the first drug approved to fight HIV—is marketed for use by people with AIDS. Although released in record time, AZT's cost—$12,000 a year—makes it the most expensive drug in history.

April

President Ronald Reagan makes his first speech about AIDS.

Oct.

"Disgusted" by safer sex comics produced by GMHC, Senator Jesse Helms introduces—and Congress passes—an amendment preventing the government from funding AIDS education that "encourages or promotes homosexual activity."

Dec. 31

59,572 cases of AIDS have been reported in the U.S.; 27,909 péople are dead.

1988　　　**Epidemic surges among women and people of color**

- Surveillance reports show that the incidence of AIDS is rising rapidly among women and people of color.

- In New York City, new AIDS cases from shared needles exceed the number of sexually transmitted new cases; and the majority of new cases are now among African Americans.

- The Alliance for Cannabis Therapeutics(ACT) receives the first inquiries from people with AIDS (PWAs) about the use of marijuana to treat the symptoms of AIDS and stimulate appetite.

Dec. 31

89,864 cases of AIDS have now been reported in the U.S.; 46,134 people are dead.

1989　　　**New drugs for people with AIDS**

- Four drugs are approved by the Food and Drug Administration (FDA) to treat illnesses associated with AIDS.

147

Aug.	A federal study indicates that AZT slows the progression of HIV infection in those who are asymptomatic or who have a few symptoms.
Sept.	Under pressure from the AIDS community, AZT's manufacturer Burroughs Wellcome lowers the price of the drug by 20%.
Nov.	The first compassionate investigational new drug (IND) request for marijuana is made by a PWA from San Antonio, Texas.
Dec. 31	115,786 cases of AIDS have been reported in the U.S.; 70,313 are dead.

1990   Landmark legislation & legal access to marijuana

Jan	The first PWA receives FDA approved supplies of marijuana for medical purposes. Steve L.'s case is reported worldwide. He dies 18 days later.
•	The Ryan White Comprehensive AIDS Resources Act (CARE) and Americans with Disabilities Act (ADA) are passed by Congress. ADA prevents discrimination against people with disabilities, including those with HIV; CARE provides disaster relief to cities and states hard hit by AIDS.
June	Dozens of health organizations from around the world protest the U.S. law barring people with HIV from entering the country by boycotting the Sixth International Conference on AIDS, held in San Francisco.
July	The first news stories about Marinol and AIDS appear. Marinol, a synthetic form of marijuana's psychoactive ingredient, has been on the market since 1986. It decreases nausea and vomiting.
Nov.	"Danny" becomes the second PWA to receive legal supplies of marijuana for medical purposes.
•	American deaths from AIDS pass the 100,000 mark. Nearly twice as many Americans have now died of AIDS as died in the Vietnam War.
Dec. 31	Three compassionate IND requests for marijuana have been filed by PWAs. One has been granted.
	161,073 cases of AIDS have been diagnosed in the U.S.; 100,813 are dead.

1991   Marijuana·AIDS Research Service is launched

Jan.

Secretary of Health and Human Services Dr. Louis Sullivan recommends that HIV infection be removed from the list of illnesses barring people with HIV from the country.

Feb. 28

The Marijuana/AIDS Research Service is launched. Barbra and Kenny Jenks become the third and fourth PWAs to receive legal marijuana.

April

Marinol, the synthetic THC pill, is granted Orphan Drug status for AIDS. Marinol sells for $8 a capsule making the average cost to an AIDS patient about $480 a month or $5760 a year.

May

The Marijuana/AIDS Research Service is represented at the 4th Annual AIDS Update Conference in San Francisco. Health professionals indicate broad support and interest in the work of MARS. PWAs become vocal about Marinol's ineffectiveness.

June

Public Health Service (PHS) moves to shut-down the FDA program of legal access to marijuana for AIDS patients citing the availability of Marinol as the reason.

•

Green Panthers shut-down HHS for over an hour in protest of the PHS decision to prohibit marijuana to AIDS patients.

July

More than 200 compassionate IND applications have been sent out by MARS. Approximately 10 have been approved.

More than 176,047 cases of AIDS have been reported in the U.S.; more than 111,815 are dead. An estimated 1,000,000 Americans are infected with HIV.

Appendix C

RESOURCES

This book is concerned only with the question of marijuana use by patients with HIV infection. The battle to legalize marijuana for medical purposes has been ongoing since 1972 and this book does not claim to adequately present the full story of that endeavour. Those seeking additional information on this topic are referred to the *Marijuana, Medicine & The Law* series from Galen Press. These books are based on court-ordered hearings before the Drug Enforcement Administration (DEA) between 1986-1988.

This book was compiled with the help of many individuals and associations. Perhaps the most remarkable aspect of the AIDS epidemic is the resourcefulness of those afflicted, the willingness to share and care. This list is barely the "tip of the iceberg." People with AIDS (PWAs) are encouraged to contact the organizations below, which will lead them to still more sources of help and information.

National Groups

Marijuana/AIDS Research Service (MARS)

A project of the Alliance for Cannabis Therapeutics (ACT), MARS was established to assist PWAs and people with HIV to obtain legal access to marijuana through the Food and Drug Administration (FDA).

> MARS
> P.O. Box 21210
> Kalorama Station
> Washington, DC 20009
> (202) 328-6391

National Association of People With AIDS (NAPWA)

NAPWA provides information on self-empowerment, education, and cooperation and interaction with local AIDS service providers to local PWA coalitions. NAPWA works to ensure that the individual and collective needs of people living with HIV infection are being met on every level.

> NAPWA
> P.O. Box 34056
> Washington, DC 20005
> (202) 898-0414

National AIDS Information Clearinghouse (NAIC)

NAIC can provide a wide range of information on AIDS, available treatments, education, and support groups.

> NAIC
> P.O. Box 6003
> Rockville, MD 20850
> (301) 762-5111

AIDS Clinical Trials Information Service (ACTIS)

ACTIS provides information on drug trials for AIDS patients and others infected with HIV. English and Spanish are spoken. Call toll free 1-800-874-2572.

National AIDS Hotline

Sponsored by the Center for Disease Control (CDC), this hotline can give you the basic facts about AIDS as well as AIDS support groups, clinics, and other services. Call toll free 1-800-342-2437. Access for Spanish speaking callers 1-800-344-7432. For the deaf 1-800-243-7889. Lines are open 7 days a week, 24 hours a day.

AIDS/HIV Experimental Treatment Directory

Published four times a year, describes drugs being tested and where the trials are being conducted. Call the American Foundation for AIDS Research (AmFAR) at (212) 719-0033.

Regional groups

ALABAMA

Ms. Sherry Wilson
Alabama Dept. of Public Health
1738 Morgan Park Dr.
Box 1059
Pelham, AL 35124
(205) 907-9259

Target Groups: Black Community, Gay/Lesbian Community, IV Drug Users, Prisoners/Parolees, Women, Youth

Services: Food Distribution, Health Care (Clinic/Walk-in), HIV Testing/Counseling (Confidential), Home Care, Pediatric AIDS Care, Physicians Referrals, Social Services, STD Testing & Treatment

ALASKA

Dr. John Middaugh
State Epidemiologist
Dept. of Health and Social Services
Epidemiology Office
3601 'C' St., Suite 540
PO Box 196333
Anchorage, AK 99519-6333

Ms. Alison King
Alaskan AIDS Assistance Assoc.
417 West 8th Avenue
Anchorage, AK 99501
(907) 276-1400 or (907) 276-4880

Services: Buddy Program, Case Management, Food Distribution, Legal Assistance, Physicians Referrals, People With AIDS Support Group, Religious Counseling/Referrals, Social Services Referrals, Volunteer Program

ARKANSAS

Dr. Ralph A. Hyman
AIDS Support Group
The Psychotherapy Center
210 Pulaski
Little Rock, AR 72201
(501) 374-3605

Target Groups: Black Community, Deaf Community, Gay/Lesbian Community, Homeless People, IV Drug Users, Women, Youth

Services: Buddy Program, Food Distribution, HIV Testing/Counseling (Anonymous), Hospice, Housing, Political Action, Physicians Referrals, People With AIDS Support Group

CALIFORNIA

Ms. Catherine Maier
San Francisco AIDS Foundation
25 Van Ness Avenue, Suite 660
San Francisco, CA 94102
(415) 864-5855

Target Groups: Asian Community, Black Community, Deaf Community, Gay/Lesbian Community, Haitian Community, Hispanic Community, Homeless People, IV Drug Users, Native American Community, Prisoners/Parolees, Women, Youth

Services: Social Services, Case Management, Food Distribution, Financial Services, Housing, Legal Assistance, People With AIDS Support Group, Social Services Referrals

Ms. Lauren Metoyer
Minority AIDS Project
5149 W. Jefferson Blvd.
Los Angeles, CA 90016
(213) 936-4949

Target Groups: Black Community, Gay/Lesbian Community, Hispanic Community, Homeless People, Native American Community, Prisoners/Parolees, Women, Youth

Services: Buddy Program, Case Management, Food Distribution, Financial Services, Home Care, Physicians Referrals, People With

AIDS Support Group, Religious Counseling/Referrals, Social Services, Social Services Referrals, Volunteer Program

Mr. Stephen Bennett
AIDS Project Los Angeles
6721 Romaine Street
Los Angeles, CA 90038
(213) 962-1600 or (800) 922-2437

Target Groups: Gay/Lesbian Community, IV Drug Users, Hispanic Community, Native American Community, Women, Youth

Services: Buddy Program, Case Management, Dental Care, Food Distribution, Home Care, Housing, Political Action, Physicians Referrals, People With AIDS Support Group, Social Services, Social Services Referrals, Volunteer Program, Legal Assistance

CONNECTICUT

Mr. William Sabella
Epidemiology Program
150 Washington Street
Hartford, CT 06106

Ms. Jean Hess
Executive Director
AIDS Project New Haven
Box 636
New Haven, CT 06503
(203) 624-0947 or (203) 624-2437

Target Groups: Black Community, Gay/Lesbian Community, IV Drug Users, Prisoners/Parolees, Women, Youth, Homeless People

Services: Buddy Program, Case Management, Food Distribution, Financial Legal Assistance, Political Action, Physicians Referrals, People With AIDS Support Group, Religious Counseling/Referrals, Social Services, Social Services Referrals, Volunteer Program

FLORIDA

Mr. Dominick Magrelli
Cure AIDS Now
2240 South Dixie Highway
Coconut Grove, FL 33133
(305) 856-8378

Services: Buddy Program, Case Management, Food Distribution, Physicians Referrals,People With AIDS Support Group, Social Services Referrals, Volunteer Program

GEORGIA

Ms. Dee Cantrell
West Central Health District
Box 2299
Columbus, GA 31993
(404) 327-1541 or (404) 323-AIDS

Target Groups: Black Community, Gay/Lesbian Community, Homeless People, IV Drug Users, Native American Community, Prisoners/Parolees, Women, Youth

Services: Buddy Program, Case Management, Food Distribution, HIV Testing/Counseling (Anonymous), HIV Testing/Counseling (Confidential), Physicians Referrals, People With AIDS Support Group, Religious Counseling/Referrals, Social Services Referrals, STD Testing & Treatment, Volunteer Program, Worried Well Support Groups

ILLINOIS

Ms. Kathy Fosdick
Central Illinois AIDS Project
1321 N. Sheridan
Peoria, IL 61606
(309) 685-8900 or (309) 685-8910

Target Groups: Gay/Lesbian Community, Women, IV Drug Users, Services: Buddy Program, Food Distribution, Physicians Referrals, People With AIDS Support Group, Social Services Referrals, Volunteer Program

IOWA

Ms. Julie Aschenbrenner
Crisis Center
321 E. First Street
Iowa City, IA 52240
(319) 351-2726 or (319) 351-0140

Services: Food Distribution, Financial Services, Physicians Referrals, Social Services Referrals, Volunteer Program, Religious Counseling/Referrals

LOUISIANA

Dr. Louise McFarland
Chief, Epidemiology Section
Louisiana Office of Preventive & Public Health Svc.
P.O. Box 60630
New Orleans, LA 70160
(504) 568-5005

Ms. Rebecca Lomax, MSW
New Orleans AIDS Project
1231 Prytania Street
New Orleans, LA 70130
(504) 523-3755

Services: Case Management, Food Distribution, Financial Services, Home Care, Hospice, Physicians Referrals, People With AIDS Support Group, Social Services Referrals, Volunteer Program

Ms. Lori LeBlanc
Coordinator
Baton Rouge AIDS Task Force
Box 66756
Baton Rouge, LA 70896
(504) 923-2277 or (504) 929-8830

Target Groups: Black Community, Gay/Lesbian Community, IV Drug Users, Women, Youth

Services: Buddy Program, Case Management, Food Distribution, Physicians Referrals, People With AIDS Support Group, Volunteer Program, Resource Library.

MAINE

William S. Nersesian, M.D.
Director, Bureau of Health
State House Station 11
Augusta, ME 04333

Perry Southerland
Director
The AIDS Project
22 Monument Square, 5th Floor
Portland, ME 04101
(207) 774-6877 or (800) 774-6877

Target Groups: Gay/Lesbian Community, Prisoners/Parolees, Deaf Community, Homeless People, IV Drug Users, Women, Youth

Services: Case Management, Food Distribution, Financial Services, HIV Testing/Counseling (Anonymous), HIV Testing/Counseling (Confidential), Political Action, Physicians Referrals, People With AIDS Support Group, Religious Counseling/Referrals, Social Services Referrals, Volunteer Program, Worried Well Support Groups

MASSACHUSETTS

Mr. Lawrence Kessler
Executive Director
AIDS Action Committee
131 Clarendon Street
Boston, MA 02116
(617) 437-6200 or (800) 235-2331

Services: Buddy Program, Case Management, Food Distribution, Financial Services, Home Care, Housing, Legal Assistance, Political Action, Physicians Referrals, People With AIDS Support Group, Religious Counseling/Referrals, Social Services, Social Services Referrals, Volunteer Program, Worried Well Support Groups

George Grady, M.D.
State Epidemiologist
Massachusetts Department of Public Health
State Laboratory Institute
305 South Street
Jamaica Plain, MA 02130
(617) 522-3700

MICHIGAN

Chief, Center for Health Promotion
3423 N. Logan
P.O. Box 30035
Lansing, Michigan 48906
(517) 373-3650 or (612) 822-7946

Target Groups: Asian Community, Black Community, Deaf Community, Gay/Lesbian Community, Hispanic Community, Homeless People, IV Drug Users, Native American Community, Prisoners/Parolees, Women, Youth

Services: Buyers' Club, Buddy Program, Case Management, Food Distribution, Home Care, Hospice, Legal Assistance, Political Action, Pediatric AIDS Care, Physicians Referrals, People With AIDS Support Group, Religious Counseling/Referrals, Social Services, Social Services Referrals, Volunteer Program, Worried Well Support Groups

Mr. Gary Rillema
Allegan County Health Dept.
2233 33rd Street
Allegan, MI 49504
(616) 673-5411

Target Groups: Gay/Lesbian Community, Hispanic Community, Women, Youth

Services: Case Management, Food Distribution, HIV Testing/Counseling (Anonymous), HIV Testing/Counseling (Confidential), Home Care, Physicians Referrals, Social Services Referrals, STD Testing & Treatment

Mr. Rick Hayner
Friends-Huron Valley
Box 7593
Ann Arbor, MI 48107
(313) 747-9068

Target Groups: Black Community, Gay/Lesbian Community, Hispanic Community, Homeless People, IV Drug Users, Women, Youth

Services: People With AIDS Support Group, Buddy Program, Food Distribution, Financial Services, HIV Testing/Counseling (Anonymous), HIV Testing/Counseling (Confidential), Home Care, Housing, Physicians Referrals, Social Services Referrals, STD Testing & Treatment, Volunteer Program, Worried Well Support Groups

MINNESOTA

Mr. Stephen Katz
Director
Aliveness Proj./PWA Coalition
730 East 38th Street
Minneapolis, MN 55407

MISSISSIPPI

Mr. Eddie Sandafer
Mississippi Gay Alliance
PWA/HIV Project
Box 8342
Jackson, MS 39284
(601) 353-7611 or (800) 537-0851

Services: Buddy Program, Case Management, Food Distribution, Financial Services, Home Care, Housing, Physicians Referrals, People With AIDS Support Group, Religious Counseling/Referrals, Social Services, Social Services Referrals, Volunteer Program.

MISSOURI

John R. Bagby, Jr, Ph.D.
Deputy Director
Environmental Health/Epidemiology Services
Missouri Department of Health
P.O. Box 570
Jefferson City, MO 65102-0570
(314) 751-8508

Mr. Gary D. Hoggard
Executive Director
AIDS Project/Springfield
309 North Jefferson, Room 254
Springfield, MO 65806
(417) 864-5607 or (417) 864-5594

Target Groups: Black Community, Gay/Lesbian Community, Homeless People, IV Drug Users, Native American Community, Prisoners/Parolees, Women, Youth

Services: Buddy Program, Case Management, Food Distribution, Financial Services, Home Care, Housing, Physicians Referrals, People With AIDS Support Group, Religious Counseling/Referrals, Social Services, Social Services Referrals, Volunteer Program, Worried Well Support Groups

Mr. Mike Flores
Heartland AIDS Resource Center
110A East 43rd Street
Kansas City, MO 64111
(816) 753-3215

Services: Food Distribution

Mr. John Hawkins
Director
Mid-Missouri AIDS Project
Box 1371
Columbia, MO 65205
(314) 875-2437

Target Groups: Black Community, Gay/Lesbian Community, Homeless People, IV Drug Users, Prisoners/Parolees, Women, Youth

Services: Buddy Program, Case Management, Dental Care, Food Distribution, Housing, Hospice, Legal Assistance, Political Action, Physicians Referrals, Volunteer Program, Religious Counseling/Referrals, Social Services Referrals

NEVADA

Ms. Sandra Ziegler
AID for AIDS of Nevada
2116 Paradise Road
Suites C & D
Las Vegas, NV 89104
(702) 369-6162

Target Groups: Gay/Lesbian Community

Services: Buddy Program, Food Distribution, Financial Services, Political Action, Physicians Referrals, People With AIDS Support Group, Social Services Referrals, Volunteer Program

NEW HAMPSHIRE

Ms. Joyce Cournoyer
Assistant State Epidemiologist
Division of Public Health Services
Bureau of Disease Control
Hlth & Welfare Bldg., Hazen Dr.
Concord, NH 03301
(603) 271-4477

NEW JERSEY

Frances Taylor, M.D.
New Jersey State Department of Health
CN 360
Trenton, NJ 08625
(609)292-7300

Jeffrey Bomser
PWAC of New Jersey
29 Grove Street
Bergenfield, NJ 07621
(201) 387-1805

Target Groups: Black Community, Gay/Lesbian Community, IV Drug Users, Women, Youth

Services: Food Distribution, People With AIDS Support Group, Worried Well Support Groups

NEW YORK

Ms. Peggy Clarke
Director, Bureau of Health Education
(212) 566-7103

or

Dr. Rand Stoneburner
Director, AIDS Surveillance and Research
(212) 566-6114
Department of Health
125 Worth St.
New York City, N.Y. 10013

Ms. Jackie Nudds
Executive Director
AIDS Rochester, Inc.
20 University Avenue
Rochester, NY 14605
(716) 232-3580 or (716) 232-4430

Services: Buddy Program, Case Management, Food Distribution, Housing, Physician Referrals, People With AIDS support group, Social Services referral, Volunteer Program, Legal Assistance, Religious Counseling Referrals, Social Services

Mr. William Case
Executive Director
PWA Coalition, Inc.
31 West 26th Street, Suite 125
New York, NY 10011
(212) 532-0290 or (212) 532-0568

Services: Food Distribution, Housing, Political Action, People With AIDS support group, Social Services, Social Services referral, Volunteer Program

Mr. Bruce Anderson
Gay Men's Health Crisis, Inc.
129 West 20th Street
New York, NY 10011
(212) 807-6664 or (212) 807-6655

Target Groups: Asian Community, Black Community, Deaf Community, Gay/Lesbian Community, Haitian Community, Hispanic

Community, IV Drug Users, Native American Community, Women, Youth

Services: Buddy Program, Case Management, Food Distribution, Financial Services, Legal Assistance, Political Action, Pediatric AIDS Care, Physician Referrals, People With AIDS support group, Social Services, Social Services referral, Volunteer Program

NORTH CAROLINA

Mr. Wilton Kennedy
Blue Ridge Health Center
Box 5151
Hendersonville, NC 28793
(704) 692-4289

Target groups: Black Community, Hispanic Community

Services: Food Distribution, Health Care (clinic/walk-in), HIV testing/counseling (anonymous), HIV testing/counseling (confidential)

OKLAHOMA

Mr. Richard E Monroe
AIDS Support Program, Inc.
2236 N.W. 39th Street
Oklahoma City, OK 73112
(405) 525-6277

Services: Buddy Program, Food Distribution, HIV testing/counseling (anonymous), People With AIDS Support Group, Referrals

OREGON

Laurence Foster, M.D.
Deputy Epidemiologist
Oregon Health Division
1400 S.W. 5th Avenue, Room 710
Portland, Oregon 97201
(503) 229-5792

C.J. Jones
President
Mid-Oregon AIDS/Support Svcs.
1115 Madison Street NE
Salem, OR 97303
(503) 363-4963

Target Groups: Gay/Lesbian Community, IV Drug Users, Prisoners/parolees

Services: Buddy Program, Food Distribution, Financial Services, Home Care, Religious Counseling referrals, Legal Assistance, Social Services, Social Services referral, Volunteer program, Physician Referral, People With AIDS Support Group, Speakers

Ms. Jeannette Bobst
Lane County Public Health
135 E. 6th Street
Eugene, OR 97401
(503) 687-4013

Services: Food Distribution, Financial Services, HIV testing/counseling (anonymous), HIV testing/counseling (confidential), Physician Referral, Social Services, STD testing & treatment

RHODE ISLAND

Mr. Phil Kane
Rhode Island Project AIDS
22 Hayes Street
Roger Williams Building
Providence, RI 02908
(401) 831-5522
(800) 726-3010

Target Groups: Gay/Lesbian Community, Hispanic Community, Black Community, IV Drug Users, Women, Youth, Native American Community

Services: Buddy Program, Case Management, Food Distribution, Financial Services, Housing, Legal Assistance, Political Action, Physician Referral, People With AIDS Support Group, Religious Counseling referrals, Social Services, Social Services referral, Volunteer program

TEXAS

Dorothy Gibson or Wesley Hodgsons
Bureau of Epidemiology
Texas Dept. of Health
1100 W. 49th St.
Austin, TX 78756
(512) 458-7328

Mr. Bernard Levy
President
AIDS Support Team
Dignity Foundation
Box 130428
Tyler, TX 75713
(214) 566-5609

Target Groups: Asian Community, Black Community, Deaf Community, Gay/Lesbian Community, Hispanic Community, Homeless people, IV Drug Users, Native American Community, Prisoners/parolees, Women, Youth

Services: Buddy Program, Case Management, Food Distribution, Financial Services, Home Care, Legal Assistance, Political Action, Pediatric AIDS Care, Physician Referral, People With AIDS Support Group, Religious Counseling referrals, Social Services, Social Services referral, Volunteer program, Worried Well support groups

Ms. Barbara Aranda-Naranjo
UT Health Science Center
7703 Floyd Curl
San Antonio, TX 78284
(512) 340-7095

Target Groups: Gay/Lesbian Community, Homeless people, IV Drug Users, Native American Community, Women, Youth

Services: Case Management, Food Distribution, Health Care (clinic/walk-in), Health Care (hospital), HIV testing/counseling (confidential), Housing, Pediatric AIDS Care, Social Services, Social Services referral, Volunteer program

Ms. Linda Patterson
Christian Community Svc. Ctr.
Box 27924
Houston, TX 77227
(713) 961-3993

Services: Food Distribution, Financial Services, Social Services referral

Mr. Valentine Rodela, Jr.
Gay & Lesbian Hispanics Unidos
Box 70153
Houston, TX 77270
(713) 520-4548

Target Groups: Hispanic Community, Gay/Lesbian Community

Services: Financial Services, Food Distribution, Social Services referral, Volunteer program

Mr. Terry D Call
Southwest AIDS Committee
916 East Yawdell
El Paso, TX 79902
(915) 533-5003 or (915) 533-6809

Target Groups: Black Community, Deaf Community, Gay/Lesbian Community, Hispanic Community, Homeless people, IV Drug Users, Prisoners/parolees, Women, Youth

Services: Buddy Program, Case Management, Food Distribution, Health Care (clinic/walk-in), HIV testing/counseling (anonymous), HIV testing/counseling (confidential), Home Care, Hospice, Housing, Legal Assistance, Political Action, Physician Referral, Religious Counseling referrals, Social Services, Volunteer program, Worried Well support groups

Jamie Shield
Education Director
AIDS Resource Center
4012 Cedar Springs
Box 190712
Dallas, TX 75219
(214) 521-5124 or (214) 522-2290

Target Groups: Gay/Lesbian Community, Youth, Women, Hispanic Community

Services: Food Distribution, HIV testing/counseling (anonymous), HIV testing/counseling (confidential), Legal Assistance, Political Action, Physician Referral, People With AIDS Support Group, Social Services referral, Volunteer program, Holistic Therapy

Ms. Janna Zumbrum
Executive Director
AIDS Services of Austin
Box 4874
Austin, TX 78765
(512) 472-2273 or (512) 472-2437

Target Groups: Deaf Community, Black Community, Hispanic Community, Gay/Lesbian Community, IV Drug Users, Women, Youth

Services: Buddy Program, Case Management, Food Distribution, Financial Services, Home Care, Housing, Legal Assistance, Pediatric AIDS Care, Physician Referral, People With AIDS Support Group, Religious Counseling referrals, Social Services, Social Services referral, Volunteer program

VIRGINIA

Mr. William Pheifer
President
Tidewater AIDS Task Force
814 West 41st Street
Norfolk, VA 23508
(804) 423-5859

Target Groups: Black Community, Gay/Lesbian Community, Homeless people, IV Drug Users, Prisoners/parolees, Women, Youth

Services: Buyers' Club, Buddy Program, Case Management, Food Distribution, Financial Services, Housing, Physician Referral, People

With AIDS Support Group, Social Services, Social Services referral, Volunteer program

WASHINGTON

Robert H. Leahy, M.D.
DSHS Division of Health
Office of Preventive Health Services
M.S. LP 174
Olympia, WA 98504
(206) 753-7520

John Kobayashi, M.D., M.P.H.
DSHS Division of Health
Office of Public Health Laboratories
  and Epidemiology
1610 N.E. 150th Street
Seattle, WA 98155-7224
(206) 367-2831

Mr. John Eric Duncan
Tacoma/Pierce County Hlth Dept
3625 South Dst. Fc3365
Tacoma, WA 98408
(206) 591-6060

Target Groups: Black Community, Deaf Community, Gay/Lesbian Community, Hispanic Community, Homeless people, IV Drug Users, Native American Community, Prisoners/parolees, Women, Youth

Services: Case Management, Food Distribution, HIV testing/counseling (anonymous), HIV testing/counseling (confidential), Political Action, Social Services referral

Ms. Tiffany Nelson
Helpers of People with AIDS
c/o ccs 1918 Everett Avenue
Everett, WA 98201
(206) 259-9188

Services: Buddy Program, Food Distribution, Volunteer program

Ms. Diane Martin
Lincoln County Health Dept.
Box 215
Davenport, WA 99122
(509) 725-1001

Target Groups: Prisoners/parolees

Services: Case Management, Food Distribution, HIV testing/counseling (anonymous), HIV testing/counseling (confidential), Physician Referral, Social Services referral

WEST VIRGINIA

Mr. Roger D. Banks
Program Coordinator
Mountain State AIDS Network
Box 1401
Morgantown, WV 26507
(304) 599-6726

Target Groups: Gay/Lesbian Community, Women, IV Drug Users, Youth

Services: Buddy Program, Case Management, Food Distribution, Physician Referral, People With AIDS Support Group, Social Services referral, Financial Services, Religious Counseling referrals, Volunteer program

WISCONSIN

Mr. Doug Nelson
Executive Director
Milwaukee AIDS Project
Box 92505
Milwaukee, WI 53202
(414) 273-2437
(800) 334-2437

Target Groups: Black Community, Gay/Lesbian Community, Hispanic Community, Homeless people, IV Drug Users, Youth, Prisoners/parolees

Services: Buddy Program, Case Management, Food Distribution, Home Care, Housing, Legal Assistance, Physician Referral, People

With AIDS Support Group, Religious Counseling referrals, Social Services referral, Volunteer program, Worried Well support groups

Ms. Patricia Eid
St. Croix Health Dept.
Box 287
Hertel, WI 54845
(715) 349-2504

Target Groups: Native American Community

Services: Case Management, Dental Care, Food Distribution, Health Care (clinic/walk-in), HIV testing/counseling (anonymous), HIV testing/counseling (confidential), Housing, Legal Assistance, Social Services, STD testing & treatment

Computer Networks

For those with a computer and modem the following services can be extremely useful.

NAPWA Online

Washington, DC

Online phone: (703) 998-3144

AIDS Bulletin Board Service

San Francisco, CA

Online phone: (415) 626-1246

Fog City Bulletin Board System

San Francisco, CA

Online phone: (415) 863-9697

Marijuana Recipes

Many PWAs would prefer not to smoke marijuana. Marijuana can be used in baking or to make tea. The following books have helpful recipes.

A Child's Garden of Grass, Jack Margolis and Richard Clorfene, Pocket Books, New York, 1970.

171

The Connoisseur's Handbook of Marijuana, William Daniel Drake, Jr., Straight Arrow Books, New York, 1971.

The Art & Science of Cooking With Cannabis, Adam Gottlieb, High Times Books, New York.

Appendix D

BIBLIOGRAPHY

The therapeutic use of marijuana by people with AIDS (PWAs) or HIV infection is very similar to the medical use of marijuana by cancer chemotherapy patients. In the early 1970s young cancer patients began reporting that marijuana greatly reduced or eliminated the dreadful nausea and vomiting caused by cancer chemotherapy. They also noted the illegal drug increased their appetites. Scientific studies later confirmed these observations. In the late 1970s and early 1980s, several states—including New Mexico, Michigan, Georgia, Tennessee, and New York—conducted state-wide programs of medical access to marijuana for victims of cancer. These state sponsored studies re-affirmed marijuana's medical utility for the treatment of cancer chemotherapy side-effects.

There have been no published studies of marijuana's therapeutic utility in the treatment of AIDS but the following bibliography of cancer studies will be useful to anyone seeking scientific readings on the subject of marijuana as an anti-nausea drug.

CANCER CHEMOTHERAPY BIBLIOGRAPHY

BOOKS

Marijuana Medical Papers, Tod Mikuriya, M.D. (ed.) Medi-Comp Press, Berkeley, California (1972).

Cannabinoids as Therapeutic Agents, Raphael Mechoulam (ed.) CRC Press, Boca Raton, Florida (1986).

Cancer Treatment & Marijuana Therapy, Robert C. Randall (ed.), Galen Press, Washington, D.C., (1990).

ARTICLES

Cancer Treatment Reports, 566:589-592, 1982.

"Cannabinoids for Nausea," *Lancet*, January 31, 1981.

Carey, M.P., Burish, T.G., & Brenner, D.E., "Delta-9-THC in Cancer Chemotherapy: Research Problems and Issues," *Annals of Internal Medicine*, 99:106-114, 1983.

Chang, A.E. *et al.*, "Delta-9-Tetrahydrocannabinol as an Antiemetic in Cancer Patients Receiving High-dose Methotrexate," *Annals of Internal Medicine*, 91:819-824, 1979.

Doblin, R.E. and Kleiman, M.A.R., "Marijuana as Antiemetic Medicine: A Survey of Oncologists Experiences and Attitudes," *Journal of Clinical Onocology*, 9:7, 1314-1319, 1991.

Harris, L., "Analgesic and Antitumor Potential of the Cannabinoids," *The Therapeutic Potential of Marijuana*, Cohen & Stillman (eds.), 299-305, 1976.

Harris, L., Munson, A. & Carchman, R., "Anti-tumor Properties of Cannabinoids," *The Pharmacology of Marihuana*, Braude & Szara (eds.), 749-762, 1976.

Neidhart, J., Gagen, M., Wilson, H. & Young, D., "Comparative Trial of the Antiemetic Effects of THC and Haloperidol," *Journal of Clinical Pharmacology*, 21:385-425, 1981.

Sallan, S.E., Zinberg, N., & Frei, E. "Antiemetic Effect of Delta-9-THC in Patients Receiving Cancer Chemotherapy," *New England Journal of Medicine*, 293:16, 795-797, 1975.

Sensky, T., Baldwin, A., & Pettingale, K., "Cannabinoids as Antiemetics," *British Medical Journal*, 286: 802, 1983.

Ungerleider, J., Andrysiak, T., *et. al.*, "Cannabis and Cancer Chemotherapy: A Comparison of Oral Delta-9-THC and Prochlorperazine," *Cancer*, 50:636-645, 1982.

Vinciguerra, Vincent, *et.al.*, "Inhalation Marijuana as an Antiemetic for Cancer Chemotherapy," *New York State Medical Journal*, 88:525-27, 1988.

GLOSSARY

A

ACT - Alliance for Cannabis Therapeutics.

Acyltransferase - Any of a group of enzymes that catalyze the transfer of an acyl group from one substance to another.

Allograft - A graft between animals of the same species, but different genotype.

AMA - American Medical Association.

Analogue - One of a group of chemical compounds similar in structure, but different in respect to elemental composition.

Anergy - Diminished reactivity to specific antigens.

Anorexia - Loss of appetite and inability to eat.

Anti-neoplastic - Destroys, inhibits, or prevents the growth or spread of neoplasms (tumors).

Antiemetic - Of or pertaining to a substance useful in suppressing nausea and vomiting.

Antigens - Any substance capable of inducing antibody formation and of reacting specifically in some detectable manner with the antibodies produced.

Arcana - Describes a pharmacologic school of thought that advocates the identification of principle active chemicals in a plant that are then synthesized for medical applications.

Armamentarium - Methods, techniques, and medications available to a physician for combatting a disease.

Aspergillosis - a disease caused by species of *Aspergillus* (a type of fungi), marked by inflammatory lesions in the skin, ears, sinuses, lungs, and sometimes bones.

Ativan™ - A brand name for lorazepam, a type of benzodiazepine, a drug commonly used to treat nervousness or tension. Other commonly known benzodiazepines include Valium™, Xanax™, and Halcion™.

Azathioprine - An antineoplastic derivative used as a cytotoxic and immunosuppressive agent in the treatment of leukemia and autoimmune diseases.

AZT - A commonly used name for zidovudine, an antiviral medication used to treat HIV infection. Common side-effects include nausea and loss of appetite.

B

Benzodiazepines - A family of drugs commonly used to treat nervousness or tension. Examples include Valium™, Xanax™, and Halcion™.

Biopsy - A process of removing tissue from the body for study and prognosis.

Blastogenesis - Morphological transformation of small lymphocytes into larger cells resembling blast cells on exposure to phytohemagglutinin or to antigens to which the donor is immunized.

BNDD - Bureau of Narcotics and Dangerous Drugs, predecessor of the DEA.

BuSpar - A brand of buspirone. Used to treat certain anxiety disorders and to relieve symptoms of anxiety.

C

Cannabinoid - Any of the chemical compounds that are the active principles of marijuana.

Cannabis - The flowering tops of the marijuana plant.

CAT scan - Computerized axial tomography (CAT). A means of scanning the human body.

Chemotherapeutic - Treatment of disease by means of chemicals that have a specific toxic effect upon disease-producing microorganisms or that selectively destroy cancerous tissues.

Chlorpromazine - A type of phenothiazine used to treat nervous, mental, and emotional disorders.

Compassionate IND - A means by which seriously ill individuals can gain access to a new drug not yet approved for marketing.

Controlled Substances Act - Federal legislation enacted in 1970 that establishes a system for regulating and controlling drugs according to certain explicit criteria. The statute established five schedules of controls for drugs. Marijuana is currently in Schedule I, the most severely restricted of the five schedules.

Cryoprecipitate - Any precipitate that results from cooling.

CSA - Controlled Substances Act of 1970.

D

Dantrium - Brand name of dantrolene, a drug used to relax certain muscles. Dantrium is used in treating multiple sclerosis (MS), cerebral palsy, stroke, or injury to the spine.

DARAC - Drug Abuse Research Advisory Committee. An advisory committee to the Food and Drug Administration (FDA) in the 1970s.

DEA - Drug Enforcement Administration.

Delta-9-THC - The psychoactive ingredient in marijuana that has been synthesized into capsule form and used for research.

Demerol - Brand name for meperidine, a narcotic analgesic used to relieve pain.

Detente - A relaxing of tensions.

ddc - An anti-HIV drug currently in Phase III testing. It belongs to the same family of drugs as AZT but appears to be more potent against the virus. Side effects may include peripheral neuropathy.

ddi - An anti-HIV drug recently approved for marketing. It has shown some promise i helping the body to increase the number of T-cell helpers but there have also been reports of high toxicity.

Dronabinol - Commercially available synthetic delta-9-THC in oral form. Used to treat nausea and vomiting following anti-cancer treatments. Brand name Marinol™.

Dyskinesia - Difficulty or abnormality in performing voluntary muscle movements.

Dysphoria - A state of dissatisfaction, anxiety, restlessness, or fidgeting. Malaise.

E

Emesis - Vomiting.

Erythrocytes - Red blood cells or corpuscles.

Euphoriant - A substance that induces euphoria — happiness, confidence, or well being.

F

Factor VIII - A protein that is essential to normal blood clotting and is deficient or lacking in people with hemophilia.

FBN - Federal Bureau of Narcotics. A federal agency that became the Drug Enforcement Administration in 1974.

FDA - Food and Drug Administration.

G

Glaucoma - An eye disease characterized by elevated intraocular pressures (IOP).

H

HIV+ - Indicates a person has tested positive for human immune deficiency disease.

Hapten - a substance having a single antigenic determinant that can react with a previously existing antibody but cannot stimulate more antibody production unless combined with other molecules; a partial antigen.

Halcion™ - Brand of benzodiazepine used to treat nervousness or tension. Also used to treat insomnia.

Hallucinations - A sensory experience of something that does not exist outside the mind, that is caused by various physical and mental disorders or by a reaction to certain substances.

Hallucinogen - A substance that causes hallucinations.

Haloperidol - A major tranquilizer of the butyrophenone series.

Hemagglutinin - An antibody that causes agglutination (clumping or massing) red blood cells.

Humoral - Of, pertaining to, or proceeding from a fluid of the body.

Hygroton - Brand of chlorthalidone, a diuretic.

I

Immunogen - Any substance or cell introduced into the body in order to generate an immune response.

Immunosuppression - The inhibition of the normal immune system because of disease, the administration of drugs, or surgery.

In limine - Latin term meaning "at the outset."

IND - Investigational new drug application. A regulatory procedure of the FDA used to test new drugs prior to approval and marketing.

Infra - Latin word meaning "below."

Inter alia - Latin phrase meaning "among other things."

In vitro - made to occur in a laboratory vessel or other controlled experimental environment rather than within a living organism or natural setting.

In vivo - occurring or made to occur within a living organism or natural setting.

K

Kaposi's Sarcoma - A cancer of connective tissue characterized by painless, purplish-red to brown plaquelike or pimply lesions on the extremities, trunk, or head.

L

LD$_{50}$ - Median lethal dose. A rating system for medications that indicates at what dosage 50% of the patients receiving the drug will die of drug-induced toxicity.

Leukocytes - Any of various nearly colorless cells of the immune system that circulate mainly in the blood and lymph and participate in reactions to invading microorganisms or foreign particles, comprising the B cells and T cells, macrophages, monocytes, and granulocytes.

Lymphocytes - A type of white blood cell having a large, spherical nucleus surrounded by a thin layer of nongranular cytoplasm.

M

Macrophage - A large white blood cell, occurring particularly in connective tissue and in the bloodstream, that ingests foreign particles and infectious microorganisms by phagocytosis.

Marijuana Tax Act - Passed in 1937, this legislation outlawed the manufacture of marijuana by severely taxing and regulating the production of the plant. It did not specifically prohibit marijuana's use in medicine, but effectively did so by creating a highly bureaucratic system that doctors quickly rejected, choosing to use more readily available synthetic drugs many of which had just been "discovered" or produced.

Marinol™ - Brand name for synthetic delta-9 THC.

Morphine - A medication used for pain relief and sedation.

Multiple Sclerosis (MS) - A chronic degenerative, often episodic disease of the central nervous system marked by patchy destruction of the myelin that surrounds and insulates nerve fibers. It usually appears in young adults and is manifested by one or more mild to severe neural and muscular impairments, as spastic weakness in one or more limbs, a local sensory loss, bladder dysfunction, or visual disturbances.

N

NAAG - National Association of Attorneys General.

NACDL - National Association of Criminal Defense Lawyers.

Naloxone - A narcotic analgesic antagonist.

NDA - New drug application. A regulatory procedure of the FDA. The NDA is applied for just prior to marketing and is the final step in the drug approval process.

Neuralgia - Sharp and paroxysmal pain along the course of a nerve.

Neuritic pain - Continuous pain in a nerve associated with paralysis and sensory disturbances.

NIDA - National Institute on Drug Abuse.

NIMH - National Institutes of Mental Health.

NORML - National Organization for the Reform of Marijuana Laws.

O

Oncology - The branch of medical science that deals with tumors, including the origin, development, diagnosis, and treatment of malignant neoplasms.

Ophthalmology - The branch of medical science that deals with the anatomy, functions, and diseases of the eye.

P

PCP - Abbreviation for *pneumocystis carinii pneumonia*, a relatively rare pneumonia. An opportunistic infection among AIDS patients.

Peripheral neuropathy - A disorder of the nerves, usually involving the feet or hands, and sometimes the legs and arms. Symptoms may include numbness, tingling or burning sensations, sharp pain, weakness, and abnormal reflexes.

Phagocytosis - The engulfing of microorganisms or other cells and foreign particles by another cell.

Pharmacopeia - A book published usually under the jurisdiction of the government that contains a list of drugs, their formulas, methods of making medicinal preparations, requirements and tests for their strength and purity, and other related information.

Phase I, II, III - Refers to the three phases of study during investigational new drug studies.

Phytohemagglutinin (PHA) - A hemagglutinin of plant origin.

Placebo - A substance that has no pharmacological effect but is administered as a control to test the efficacy of a medicinal agent.

Prednisone - A cortisone-like medicine used to provide relief for inflamed areas of the body.

Protocol - The plan for carrying out a scientific study or a patient's treatment regimen.

Psychoactive - A substance that has a profound or significant effect on mental processes.

Psychopharmacology - The branch of pharmacology that deals with the psychological effects of drugs.

Psychotropic - A drug, such as a tranquilizer, sedative, or anti-depressant, that affects mental activity, behavior, or mood.

Psychotomimetic - Psychosis-like.

S

Sublethal - Almost lethal or fatal.

Self-titrate - Occurs when the patient is able to determine the proper and appropriate dosage of medicine. When used in this book, self-titrate usually refers to the advantage of inhaled marijuana over oral antiemetic medications.

Spasm - A sudden, abnormal, involuntary muscular contraction.

Spasticity - A condition characterized by sudden, abnormal, involuntary muscular contraction or a series of alternating muscle contractions and relaxations.

Schedule I, II - Two of the five classifications in the Controlled Substances Act. Schedule I and II have basically the same definition with the exception that Schedule I drugs have "no accepted medical value in the United States."

SSI - Supplemental Security Insurance. A disability insurance program operated by the Social Security Administration.

T

T-cells - Any of several closely related lymphocytes developed in the thymus, that circulate in the blood and lymph and orchestrate the immune system's response to infected or malignant cells.

Tincture - A solution of alcohol or of alcohol and water, that contains animal, vegetable, or chemical drugs.

Tachycardia - Excessively rapid heartbeat.

THC - Tetrahydrocannabinol is the major psychoactive ingredient in marijuana. In most instances this refers to delta-9-THC.

Thrush - A disease characterized by whitish spots and lesions on the membranes of the mouth. Caused by parasitic fungus.

Titration - Sufficient intake of a substance to create a recognizable therapeutic action.

V

Veteran's Administration (VA) - A federal agency charged with caring for and administering programs for America's military veterans.

W

Wasting syndrome - A condition characterized by involuntary weight loss of more than 10% of baseline body weight plus either chronic diarrhea or chronic weakness and fever for more than 30 days, when these conditions cannot be explained by other than HIV infection.

INDEX

V

VA Hospital, 135

U

U.S. Court of Appeals, 10

W

Warner, Senator John, 67
Wasting syndrome, 13

Y

Young, Francis   6, 71

about the author

Robert Randall is one of the nation's leading experts on marijuana's medical use. Mr. Randall is afflicted with glaucoma—a blinding eye disease. In 1976, he made legal and medical history when the courts ruled his use of marijuana was not criminal, but an act of "medical necessity." He obtained legal access to federally-produced supplies of marijuana in that same year. As Randall puts it, "Uncle Sam became my dealer."

Randall, who continues to receive marijuana-by-prescription, has become a leading advocate for medical access to marijuana for the treatment of life- and sense-threatening diseases. In 1980, he founded the Alliance for Cannabis Therapeutics, a non-profit, patients-rights organization. He continues to serve as ACT's president and chief spokesperson. He has lectured extensively in the United States and Europe and written for publications as diverse as the *Washington Post, Playboy, High Times* and the *Journal on Addiction Research.* He has appeared on all major national television news shows, "Good Morning America," "Larry King Live," "Today," and even "To Tell The Truth."

Mr. Randall has edited four books in the series *Marijuana, Medicine & The Law.* These books, based on extensive hearings before the Drug Enforcement Administration (DEA), constitute the most complete examination of marijuana's medical use in the 20th century.

other books from Galen Press

Marijuana, Medicine & The Law, Volume I : The Direct Testimony
ISBN: 0-936485-02-7. 502 pages, softcover, $29.95

"The specific nature of this collection is to be commended . . . a solid piece of research." That's what the *Midwest Book Review* said of this first volume. Detailed affidavits from more than fifty-five witnesses, including many of the world's leading medical experts on marijuana's therapeutic uses, patients, scientists, researchers, attorneys, and health administrators.

Marijuana, Medicine & The Law, Volume II: The Legal Argument
ISBN: 0-936485-04-3. 484 pages, softcover. $25.95

Volume II transforms the vast body of evidence into concise, thoroughly documénted, and easy-to-read legal arguments.Includes the legal briefs from the DEA and the petitioning parties as well as selected portions of the oral arguments. The full text of Chief DEA Administrative Law Judge 's historic ruling —which concludes marijuana has significant therapeutic benefits—is reprinted. The extensive bibliography and numerous exhibits makes this book a valuable reference tool.

Cancer Treatment & Marijuana Therapy
ISBN: 0-936485-05-1. 365 pages. Softcover. $23.95

"[T]his book raises important questions about the bureaucratic process and our political, judicial, and medical systems." That's what *Oncology Nursing Forum* said about *Cancer Treatment & Marijuana Therapy*. In addition to the compelling testimony of witnesses, this book also contains the recently published survey of American oncologists conducted by Harvard University which reveals that 70% favor prescriptive access to marijuana. Data from unpublished state research programs makes this book particularly valuable. The book is fully indexed with a glossary of terms.

Muscle Spasm, Pain & Marijuana Therapy
ISBN: 0-936485-06-X. 237 pages. Softcover. $14.95

"Almost everyone in the [paralyzed] community has heard this helpful home tip for controlling muscle spasms: smoke marijuana." *Spinal Network Extra*. This release from Galen Press documents the widespread use of marijuana by individuals with paralysis, multiple sclerosis, and spinal injury to control often debilitating muscle spasms. The book also documents the use of marijuana in treating chronic pain from arthritis and other ailments.

Galen Press, P.O. Box 53318, Washington, DC 20009
(202) 462-3080.
Individual orders must be prepaid. Major credit cards accepted.